Praise for *How Do You Choose?*

"This book is a gift. If you've ever been curious about who you truly are and how you're designed to move through the world, this is your guide. With clarity and depth, Erin Claire Jones illuminates the wisdom of Human Design, helping you unlock your innate strengths, release what's not yours to carry, and step into a life of ease and alignment. Erin's wisdom has changed my life, and I'm certain it can change yours, too."

—Amber Rae, bestselling author of *Choose Wonder Over Worry*

"When this book arrived at my doorstep, I felt it was a sign from the Universe. Erin eloquently explains the intricacies of Human Design and how to integrate this system into your everyday life. I absolutely adore this book!"

—Gabby Bernstein, #1 *New York Times* bestselling author

"I wish I had *How Do You Choose?* years ago! Erin Claire Jones takes the guesswork out of decision making and helps you trust your own path. This isn't just another personality test—it's a roadmap to making choices that actually fit you. Packed with insights and real-life strategies, this book will help you move with confidence toward the life you're meant to live."

—Jenna Kutcher, *New York Times* bestselling author and educator

"As a seasoned astrologer, I have always been fascinated by personality types. Human Design has called my name, but it wasn't until Erin Claire Jones's book that the system truly clicked. She teaches like I teach—through storytelling, real-life examples, and clear, accessible language.

If Human Design has ever felt like a tangle of jargon, *How Do You Choose?* will ground it in everyday life. It bridges the gap between spirituality and practicality, making this powerful tool feel relevant, approachable, and deeply useful."

—Debra Silverman, MA, astrologer, psychotherapist, and author

"*How Do You Choose?* isn't just a book—it's a personalized blueprint to living your best life. It's about achieving greater success, creating meaningful, lasting connections, and making decisions with ease. Imagine a life where you thrive in every area—this is your first step toward that transformation."

—Jay Shetty, #1 *New York Times* bestselling author and host of the *On Purpose* podcast

"The roadmap to understanding yourself you didn't know you needed. Erin Claire Jones makes Human Design practical, relatable, and easy to apply—whether you're looking to improve your relationships, find more fulfillment in your work, or simply move through life with greater clarity. Insightful, empowering, and full of 'aha' moments, it's the kind of book you'll want to revisit again and again."

—Vienna Pharaon, national bestselling author of *The Origins of You*

HOW DO YOU CHOOSE?

A
HUMAN DESIGN
GUIDE TO
WHAT'S BEST FOR YOU
AT WORK, IN LOVE,
AND IN LIFE

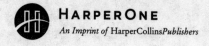
HarperOne
An Imprint of HarperCollins*Publishers*

HOW DO YOU CHOOSE?

Erin Claire Jones
Founder of Human Design Blueprint

HarperCollins books may be purchased for educational, business, or sales promotional use. For information, please email the Special Markets Department at SPsales@harpercollins.com.

FIRST EDITION

Library of Congress Cataloging-in-Publication Data has been applied for.

ISBN 978-0-06-341277-4

25 26 27 28 29 LBC 5 4 3 2 1

To my clients, students, and community—
thank you for sharing your stories and selves
so generously with me over the years, and for
teaching me more about Human Design than any
class ever could.

All I can do is be me, whoever that is.

—BOB DYLAN

Contents

3 Authority 141

How You Make Decisions

HOW DO YOU CHOOSE?

Introduction

IN 2015 I WAS TWENTY-FOUR YEARS OLD, LIVING IN NEW YORK CITY, and working for an early-stage financial tech company. After only two years in the trenches of start-up life, I was in the midst of a genuine quarter-life crisis. Romantically, I was navigating an on-again, off-again relationship. Professionally, part of me wanted to enter venture capital, and another wanted to build an essential oils business. A third part of me wanted to sell my belongings and move to Bali.

One night, I went to a party on Manhattan's Lower East Side, struck up a conversation with a friend of a friend, and found myself sharing details about my prolonged indecision.

"Have you ever heard of Human Design?" he asked me.

"Of course," I said, assuming he was referencing human-centered design, a popular approach to product development believed to have been created at Stanford University. But when he asked for my time, date, and place of birth, I realized we weren't discussing how to choreograph user experiences. Instead, he used my details to generate a digital chart of intricate lines, numbers, and shapes. After analyzing my chart, he shared reflections of me that felt eerily spot-on.

"You're meant to be a teacher and a guide," he said. "And you're not supposed to work so hard all the time. Your talent is making people feel seen and asking the right questions. Life should be a bit more flowy for someone like you."

Introduction

His words washed over me like a cool breeze. While being curious about people and asking questions were undoubtedly my gifts—my parents always thought I'd be a therapist—I had never considered those gifts valuable enough to build a career around. They were simply part of me; they always had been.

"How do you know that about me?" I asked in disbelief, grasping for his phone. "What else does that thing say?"

"You're a Projector," he said. "You're meant to lead by offering perspective and to work in short sprints with lots of rest in between."

I asked him what a Projector was.

"It's one of the five Types in Human Design."

It sounded like science fiction. But it also sounded . . . well . . . accurate.

He explained that Human Design is a modality for self-understanding, like astrology, the Enneagram, or Myers-Briggs. Like astrology, it draws on a person's time, date, and place of birth to generate a chart that reveals their core personality characteristics. Like the Enneagram, it unlocks insights into how they can find their flow in relationships and at work. And like Myers-Briggs, Human Design explains under what conditions people feel most energized and empowered.

Beyond my being a Projector, he shared two additional pieces of my Human Design that would help me navigate big questions about love and work.

The first was called my Strategy. He explained that in Human Design, your Strategy is the way you're designed to cultivate opportunities.

"And *your* Strategy," he said, "is to Wait for an Invitation. It means you should wait to be invited into opportunities or relationships rather than pounding the pavement trying to initiate them yourself."

I pushed back. "That can't be right. I pursued my current job, and that is the only way anything has ever happened for me."

"And how's that feeling?" he asked.

Reflecting on his question, I was clearly burning the candle at both ends, which wasn't just exhausting—it was unsustainable. Yet I hadn't found another way to strive for success.

"How does it feel when you think about waiting for invitations to share your gifts instead of pushing so hard to force opportunities?" he asked.

"Honestly, it feels like a relief, but also a little scary and hard to trust."

His last insight was about my decision-making process, which he called my Authority.

"You have an Emotional Authority," he said. "This means you're not meant to make decisions quickly, and you should avoid drawing conclusions on emotional highs and lows."

For example, if I am excited about a new job, I should wait a few days until my emotions settle before deciding whether to take it. Or if I'm feeling down about a relationship, it's best to move through my feelings before making a rash decision and calling it quits. Essentially, I should give myself time and space to process before making big decisions.

I felt more recognized with every insight he shared. I began to understand why the approaches that seemed to work for other people—like initiating new ideas and businesses, being uberproductive, and making quick decisions—didn't work for me.

I *was* working too hard. I *was* burning out often. I barely got enough sleep at night let alone breaks during the day. I chased after opportunities to no avail. I made decisions quickly and often regretted them. I knew I had a talent for seeing the big picture and making people feel seen, but my work wasn't structured around these gifts.

For the rest of the evening, he explained how I could use those Human Design elements—Type, Strategy, and Authority—to choose what was best for me at work, in love, and in life.

When I got home that night, I must have read a hundred articles about Human Design, Projectors, how to Wait for an Invitation, Emotional Authorities, and honestly, how to know when a con artist has duped you. My mind was blown. And if Human Design wasn't mysterious enough, its origin story was even more fantastic.

As the legend goes, in 1987, Alan Krakower, a middle-aged Canadian advertising executive who had uprooted his life and moved to Ibiza, was walking home one evening when he heard a voice that whispered, "It's time to work." Over the following eight days, he conceived of the Human

Design system and called it the "science of differentiation." Soon after, he changed his name to Ra Uru Hu and shared his teachings far and wide until his untimely death in 2011.

Does this sound like something out of the Marvel Cinematic Universe? You bet. But when I looked under the hood at Alan's—er, Ra's—creation, it seemed quite remarkable.

Human Design couples NASA planetary data with the zodiac, the I Ching, and Eastern philosophy to generate a chart that explains how energy moves through our bodies, what types of people and opportunities are best for us, what our strengths and challenges are, and so much more. It sits at the intersection of spirituality and practicality, offering a fun, mystical approach to living our most productive, connected lives.

As I delved deeper into Human Design, I noticed that the system offered two benefits I hadn't yet experienced across various personality assessments. The first was a useful framework for understanding myself and my relationships, providing a language for our differences. For instance, learning that I was a Projector who wasn't built to burn the midnight oil and my friend was a Manifesting Generator, a type that typically has more energy than a college fraternity, was revelatory. It helped me appreciate her capacity to go, go, go, while also learning to communicate my own desire to sometimes linger behind and enjoy a quiet moment with a book.

Second, Human Design gave me practical tools to transform my life immediately. Often, with personality assessment tools, we receive powerful information about ourselves but can struggle to apply it meaningfully. With Human Design, that wasn't the case. Almost immediately, I started building breaks into my days, investing more energy in places where I felt seen, and avoiding making decisions during emotional highs or lows. I allowed myself time to process and choose what was best for me without concession.

Within six months of discovering my Human Design, my feelings of indecision were gone, and I knew exactly what my next moves should be. As someone designed to be a guide and teacher who succeeds far more through invitation than initiation and who needs to be fully emotionally regulated before making serious decisions, I decided to be entirely single, leave my job, move to Bali, support myself through Airbnb, and study Human Design full-time. Did this feel irresponsible? A little. Given an Ivy League education and a burgeoning start-up career, did it make sense? Not entirely. But did it feel like the best thing for me? Absolutely.

Within a year of that fateful night in New York City, I offered readings and produced hyperpersonalized guides that I called "blueprints" for friends and acquaintances. These guides provided actionable insights into how a person could show up more fully at work, in love, and in life according to their unique design.

Ten years later, my company, Human Design Blueprint, has introduced Human Design to more than five hundred thousand people through social media and my blog. We have generated over a million Human Design charts for people across 160 countries, produced more than forty thousand personalized guides, and trained more than a thousand Human Design teachers—many of whom now have thriving practices of their own.

I have shared insights globally at corporate giants and small companies alike and have done one-on-one sessions for over three thousand people, including orchestra conductors, professional basketball players, executives, ceramicists, pastry chefs, heart surgeons, psychiatrists, full-time parents, and everyone in between. I have laughed with them, cried with them, and relished those magical moments when I see the ineffable look on their faces, screaming, "I feel seen!"

My nondogmatic belief in Human Design and its application in our lives has always set me apart from other Human Design professionals. As someone who followed a more traditional academic path, the question I've grappled with from the beginning of my Human Design journey has always been: Does the information have to be *true* to be *helpful*? Put differently: What *practical* roles can mysticism and spirituality play in our lives?

I've found that regardless of how far-fetched or uncanny these insights may seem, they offer us an opportunity to jump-start a meaningful internal conversation about who we are and what we choose.

Like all my clients, I discovered Human Design at a crossroads, asking myself, *Should I do this or that? How do I choose what's best?* Perhaps that's where you are now. Maybe you're wondering if a relationship is right for you, if you should change lanes in your career, or if you should move to a new city. For all these decisions and more, this book offers you an inspiring new pathway to self-discovery, clarity, and power.

How to Use This Book

The book is divided into three sections: Type, Strategy, and Authority, the same elements of Human Design that changed my life. Admittedly, these sections merely skim the surface of what Human Design can offer, but they're the best place to begin for anyone looking to make immediate and meaningful shifts. Collectively, they reveal how to use your energy most effectively, how to find and create the right opportunities, and how to make the best decisions.

In each chapter, I'll offer insights into how that particular element is expressed and the ways it can empower you in relationships and at work. I'll also suggest practical ways to integrate it into your life. Every chapter will begin with a celebrity whose chart includes this aspect and explore how it may have shown up in their life. While these stories have been chosen based on the most accurate birth time of each person available, exact times can be uncertain, so take these stories as illustrative rather than definitive.

In the first section, we'll explore the five Types. You'll discover who has nonstop energy, works best in waves, is meant to guide, and kickstarts big ideas. You'll learn how a small-town chef used her Type to make the bold decision to close up shop and cook on the front lines in Ukraine, how a daughter estranged from her father used her Type to make amends, and how a married couple headed for divorce used their Types to save their relationship.

In the second section, we'll explore the four Strategies. You'll learn who should go after what they want and who should let things come to them. You'll meet a burned-out surgeon who used her Strategy to make a career pivot, a single woman who used her Strategy to break a dating dry spell, and a marketer who used her Strategy to pump the brakes on a lucrative career and dive headfirst into a new passion.

In the final section, we'll explore the seven Authorities. You'll find out who should trust their gut in the moment and who should sleep on big decisions. You'll discover why some people need to talk decisions out amongst friends, while others find clarity in solitude. You'll learn how a bride used her Authority to call off her wedding and head back to school, how a disillusioned surfer used his Authority to get back on the board, and how a single woman at a café used her Authority to identify the stranger who would become her life partner.

Look Up Your Design

Before you dive in, go to humandesignblueprint.com and look up your Human Design. Take note of your Type, Strategy, and Authority.

To generate your chart, you'll need your time, date, and place of birth. If you're unsure of your exact time of birth, use the closest approximate you know. If you only know the day or a general time (like morning or afternoon), try looking up a few times within that range to see if your Type or Authority changes. This is usually consistent, but it can vary. If you find differences, you can review the possibilities in the book to see which resonates most. For birthplace, the location is used to determine the time zone you were born in, so if you don't know the precise city, simply choose a region within the correct time zone.

It's important to note that, while each section covers *all* the Types, Strategies, and Authorities, only one chapter from each section will explicitly be about *your* Type, Strategy, and Authority. For instance, my Type is Projector, my Strategy is Wait for an Invitation, and my Authority is Emotional. This is why I also recommend looking up the designs of one or two other people in your life—perhaps your partner, sibling, parent, child, or colleague.

Once you have the designs of the people you love in hand, the other chapters will help you better understand and engage with them. My husband's Type is Generator, his Strategy is Wait to Respond, and his Authority is Sacral. Knowing these elements of his design has transformed our relationship, allowing me to support him in a way that truly resonates with who he is.

Time to Tune In

As I was leaving that party in New York City, my new, mysterious friend shared one final thought.

"Maybe you should teach this stuff," he suggested, sensing both my enthusiasm and the relief I felt in learning my own design.

Within days, he became my first mentor and shared dozens of Human Design recordings and teachings with me. He invited me to sit in on sessions with clients and eventually let me take the lead. Without his invitation that night—remember, my Strategy is to Wait for an Invitation—I wouldn't be on this path.

When we tune into our designs, whether we're meant to wait for invitations or initiate everything ourselves, whether we have all the energy in the world or require lots of rest along the way, whether we know what's best in the moment or need to wait thirty days before making a big decision, we are empowered to live our best lives.

Know that Human Design is one of many ways to think about your personality, relationships, career, and purpose. This book may have some ideas that fully resonate with you and others that don't feel true. I encourage you to take what feels useful and leave the rest behind. The way I see it, life is rife with challenges and uncertainty. Why not take all the support we can get?

1

Type

How You Use Your Energy Best

- Your Type reveals your strengths and needs.

- It offers insights about how to manage your energy daily, how to tap into your gifts at work, how to find fulfillment in your relationships, how to be crystal clear about your needs with those you love, and how to collaborate effectively with others.

- The five Types are Generators, Manifesting Generators, Projectors, Manifestors, and Reflectors.

PERCENT OF POPULATION	36
TRADEMARK	Passion
GIFTS	Bringing ideas to life, inspiring others with your passion, completing tasks skillfully, mastering your chosen field
CHALLENGES	Being so capable and energetic that you fill your time with mundane tasks at the cost of your passions, feeling guilty about dedicating time to what you love, trying to do everything yourself, struggling with boundaries, expecting others to do as much as you
POPULAR ROLES	Entrepreneur, specialist, software engineer, researcher, artisan, chef, artist, author, teacher, speaker, consultant, athlete
RELATIONSHIP NEEDS	Space to explore your interests, respect for your boundaries, consideration of what you truly have the energy for, supportive environment to ask for help, relief from tasks that drain you, thoughtful questions about what excites you

Generator

WITH JUST TEN SECONDS LEFT IN THE THIRD QUARTER AGAINST the Oklahoma City Thunder, LeBron James stepped back and sank his thirty-sixth point of the night. The crowd erupted as James paused to take in the moment and smiled at the thousands who had come to witness history. He had officially become the highest-scoring player of all time.

The previous record, set nearly forty years earlier by NBA legend Kareem Abdul-Jabbar, was long considered unbreakable.

Yet in his twentieth season with the NBA, James broke it. How did he do it? Unlike many players known for a single iconic shot or play, James's greatness lies in his consistency, passion, and stamina.

Reflecting on his journey, James shared, "I've always wanted to be one of the greatest to ever play the game. I knew I was born with some gifts . . . but that only gets you so far. . . . So I just had to put the work into it." His lifelong passion for basketball and willingness to work harder than anyone else set him apart.

LeBron James perfectly embodies the traits of his type, a Generator: steady, energetic, passionate, dedicated, and always striving for mastery.

How Do You Choose?

At Work

As a Generator, you make things happen. When you feel genuinely excited about your work, your energy knows no bounds. You're dedicated, meticulous, and enjoy the step-by-step process of turning an idea into reality. Generators are steady, reliable, and full of life.

This means that doing what you love is not a selfish choice; to the contrary, it's one of the most generous choices you can make. When you feel satisfied by your work, your passion fills the room and your enthusiasm brings others to life too. People can't help but want to be around your bright, uplifting energy. However, when you focus your attention on tasks that feel misaligned and draining, your Generator magic quickly dissipates, and your frustration is felt by your collaborators. A Generator who is enthusiastic about what they're working on is a gift to the world. Poet Walt Whitman said it best: "Some people are so much sunshine to the square inch."

The Generators in my life have proven to be some of the most dependable and joyful people to work with. In fact, whenever I start something new, I make a conscious effort to have a Generator by my side. Collaborating is a pleasure because they bring consistent energy and a contagious passion to their work. When I feel unmotivated and depleted, they are the ones who inspire me to keep going—provided they're fulfilled by what they're working on.

It's important as a Generator to have strong boundaries at work. You possess such powerful energy that people might sense your capacity and ask you to handle anything and everything. You might also believe you should do something just because you can, and so you take on every task, burning yourself out in the process. Notice when you find yourself overextended or saying yes out of a sense of obligation or the desire to please. Learning to say no is a necessary skill. If that feels difficult or unnatural, consider this: no one benefits when you say yes simply because you think you should. In fact, saying yes without energy or conviction only leads to burnout. When you focus *primarily* on the tasks that bring you satisfaction at work, you will have more energy and less stress, and invigorate your collaborators.

The key word is *primarily*. We all have mundane but essential tasks we must do, such as responding to emails, handling administrative work, or filing taxes. What's important is that your schedule isn't exclusively filled with these duties, and that time and space are created for activities that bring you genuine satisfaction on a daily basis. The goal is not to be 100 percent lit up by everything you do, but to feel primarily gratified. Prioritizing this will give you more energy to do everything else. Some of my clients prefer a less demanding job that pays the bills but allows time for their passions on the side. One client chose an analyst support role with predictable hours so she could write her novel in her free time; in her words, "It is the work that brings me satisfaction, that lights up my energy for me, and no one else."

As a Generator, you also have a natural potential for depth. Your sustained energy and enthusiasm make you likely to immerse yourself in subjects and to master them, just as LeBron James did with basketball.

Understand that your ability to dive deep and consistently make things happen is a gift not everyone possesses. Expecting others to share your drive for mastery and excellence or your level of stamina can lead to frustration. Take the time to discover the distinct talents of those around you rather than assuming they can or should work just like you.

In an optimal role as a Generator, you have room to immerse yourself in something you're passionate about. Your day-to-day tasks bring you fulfillment. Both your work and colleagues inspire and energize you. You maintain boundaries that prevent you from biting off more than you can chew, and you are not expected to handle everything yourself. You can delegate or collaborate with others on tasks that consistently exhaust you. One of those people may be a Projector who is attuned to your energy and knows exactly what needs to be taken off your plate, or a fellow Generator or Manifesting Generator who is avid about an aspect of the process that you are not. Your team takes the initiative to free up your energy, allowing you to focus on the activities that bring you satisfaction. They are happy to do this because they innately understand that being around a lit-up Generator is galvanizing, whereas being around a depleted Generator is rapidly draining.

You know you are on track when you wake up excited to tackle the problems ahead and experience profound satisfaction at day's end, dropping into bed delightfully spent, knowing you've left it all on the field. Using your energy well is the key to deep sleep and fulfilling days—and ultimately, a satisfying life.

If you are consistently frustrated at work or feel restless and struggle to sleep, it's a sign that something may need to shift and that you're not yet using your energy in a rewarding way. While occasional frustration is a natural part of work and life, persistent dissatisfaction and restlessness are a call to consider whether your work truly offers the joy you crave.

While you may be competent at many things as a Generator, the path that ignites your passion and brings you satisfaction is the right one for you. It's not simply the destination that matters; the journey itself should feel just as gratifying.

Soul Food

Matisse and I held our session in her sunlit kitchen. I could tell this was her sanctuary, but her green eyes lacked a liveliness I sensed had once been there. My suspicion was confirmed when Matisse confided that she was feeling unsure of her next step at work. She ran a successful catering business, which she felt *should* be a dream come true for a seasoned chef like herself. And at first, it had been a dream come true. Matisse's client roster expanded quickly, and she hired a team to support her flourishing business. But over time, Matisse found that her days, once filled with inventing recipes, were now consumed by spreadsheets, meetings, managing employees, and navigating the emotional roller coaster of clients with ever-changing minds. She was burned out.

"My work used to feel like my purpose," she sighed. "Now it feels like the bane of my existence. What am I supposed to do?"

"Do you still feel inspired by cooking?" I asked.

Matisse's response was enthusiastic. "Absolutely. Yes!"

"And does managing a company energize you in the same way?"

"Not even a little bit," she responded without pause.

There it was: the truth of the matter. Whenever Matisse spoke about cooking, she lit up. But when the topic shifted to managing her business, she contracted. She wasn't worn out from cooking too much but too *little*. The countless hours of administrative tasks associated with running a small business chipped away at her energy and, ultimately, her desire to be in the food service industry at all.

"Are you building a catering business because it feels like the right path for you?" I asked. "Or because you think you should?"

I saw recognition spread across Matisse's face as she realized that her career, which had been rooted in passion, now felt like an obligation.

So often, Generators like Matisse find themselves sacrificing their own satisfaction in pursuit of what they think they *should* do. They believe they should put their powerful energy to work serving everyone else's needs or treading the expected path. Yet deprioritizing their own passion only serves to deplete a Generator's energy and puts them on a fast track to burnout. Feeling personally satisfied at work is *the* crucial piece that energizes Generators and fuels their ability to have a big, positive impact on the world.

Inspired by our session and with full permission to put her own needs on the front burner, Matisse decided to close her catering company, return to her previous career as a private chef, and focus on what she did best: cooking. She was terrified to shut down a successful business for an unknown future, but it felt right and enlivening, so Matisse trusted that. She was rewarded for trading a life filled with tedious meetings and paperwork for one dedicated to two of her big loves—cooking and creativity. Reengaged in what she loved, the energy, excitement, and fuel for her craft surged back.

Months later, Matisse sent an email that brought me to tears. Her private chef business was thriving. She felt fulfilled by how she was spending her days, and her clients shared how much they enjoyed working with someone who poured so much love into their work. But there was more! As a Ukrainian, Matisse felt called to help in whatever way she could when the war broke out in 2022. Working as a private chef allowed her the time and resources to return to her home country and cook for those on the front lines. She no longer felt misguided for following what felt right over what she thought she should do. She moved forward confidently with the knowledge that feeling personally enriched by her work was the surest path to benefiting the people and world around her.

In Relationships

As a Generator, you have the potential to elevate the joy, excitement, and passion in any relationship. Think of yourself like a hot-air balloon. When your fire is lit, you soar high, expanding and lifting everyone around you.

Yet I often see Generators burdened with a disproportionate amount of responsibility in relationships—managing household tasks, parenting duties, and work commitments, all while neglecting their own passions and having little time for themselves. In cases like this, the Generator ends up burned out and exhausted, feeling taken advantage of and resentful toward those they love. This is why it's important as a Generator to choose relationships where you feel recognized for all you do without being expected to do everything yourself.

As someone who is married to a Generator, I've seen firsthand how easy it is to rely on them because they are so capable. My husband is incredibly energetic and adept at getting things done—a true powerhouse—and it's tempting to expect him to handle it all: juggling balls at work and caring for our animals and children at home. However, eventually, even the most resourceful Generators—like my husband—reach a breaking point and feel used. Human Design has taught me that just because he *can* do something doesn't mean he *should*. Knowing this has helped me remember (most of the time) not to expect him to do it all, and to be intentional about creating space for the activities that animate him. His most passionate, excited self energizes all of us.

For those of us who love Generators, it is essential to recognize this dynamic early on in relationships. We can support our Generators by not expecting them to shoulder every responsibility, by easing their load to free up space for their interests, by taking the time to understand their energy limits, and by respecting their yeses and nos. Simple, direct questions like "Do you want to do this?" or "Does the timing feel right for this?" can help us understand what they truly have the energy for.

One client realized that the key to improving her relationship with her Generator husband was to stop forcing activities he disliked. Another Generator noted that feeling acknowledged in his desires was incredibly healing and addressed a deep-seated feeling that his needs were overlooked. Another client, a Generator who is married to a Generator, shared that their love language is giving each other permission to engage in pursuits that bring them joy and center them. Her husband might say, "I'll take the kids. Go write. I can tell you want to!" Or she might hand her husband his jacket and tell him, "You need time in the yard. I can feel it."

I once advised a Generator who had been a stay-at-home mom for five years. She adored her four children but also felt a strong pull to return to work and tap into her intellectual and professional gifts. This desire ignited a sense of overwhelming guilt. I encouraged her to explore part-time work despite this internal conflict, explaining that the more energized she felt, the more positivity she would bring into her home. It wasn't until she hired a part-time nanny and dipped her toe back into work that she started to believe me. Her energy levels surged, and she saw a difference not only in herself but also in her children—everyone was lighter, brighter, and happier. It's important that Generator parents pursue what moves them, even when it doesn't include their kids. When you're energized, you uplift your children, and you may even find it easier to handle tasks that aren't as inspiring.

Many of the Generators I work with fail to recognize how their energy can set the tone for those around them. When you are excited about how you use your energy daily, it renders you a delightful, motivating presence for your friends, partner, and family. If you are frustrated and feel weighed down by your job or commitments, that discontent spills out into the home too, which makes you more likely to suck the energy out of a room.

This means as a Generator, having space in a relationship to pursue your passions, whether independently or with others, and to freely share what you're working on and thinking about is essential. It can feel disheartening when you're eager to share something you're passionate about—like your newfound interest in Human Design—but those around you seem disinterested. You thrive when your loved ones are curious about what's engaging your energy and ask thoughtful questions about what you're working on.

You might also find you have more energy than your partner or friends, which can make it difficult for them to keep pace with you. Over the course of hundreds of couples sessions, I've observed that much of the disappointment in relationships for Generators is rooted in the expectation that others will operate similarly. Maybe a partner expects you to spend a lazy Sunday at home, but you prefer to work on your music or garden. Or you might feel disappointed if a loved one can't match your energy levels or wants to take a break from a project you adore. Often, the issue isn't with your relationship; it's simply a gap in understanding. Just like in work, it's important to recognize your differences and understand that not everyone can keep up with you—nor are they meant to.

For example, whenever my Generator husband and I arrive in a new city, his first instinct is to drop off our bags and start exploring, while mine is to lie down and recharge after a long day of travel. I used to push myself to keep up with him—like the time we arrived in Italy, and I nearly fell asleep on the curb while he eagerly bounced in and out of every shop. Now when we land in a new city, he adventures while I rest. He honors his pace and I honor mine.

Differences in energy levels can even show up in your nighttime routines. Generators typically sleep best after fully expending their energy throughout the day, whereas other Types might prefer getting into bed earlier, before they're completely tired out. Instead of conforming to a partner's sleep schedule, make sure to prioritize your need to fully exert your energy. This could involve working late, doing a nighttime workout, or taking a walk—anything that helps you use up that last bit of energy.

As a Generator, your relationships should make you feel satisfied—at least most of the time. Relationships that regularly cause frustration may need more attention or a shift, such as setting new boundaries or temporarily stepping away to consider if a lasting change is needed. As poet Rupi Kaur put it, "i do not need the kind of love / that is draining / i want someone / who energizes me."

Lost and Found

Alice used to feel vibrant and passionate, but that now seemed like a distant memory. By the time we met, she was run-down and wondering if she would ever find her way back to herself again. As if that wasn't enough, she was also struggling in her relationship with her husband, Jack. Alice came to me questioning whether her marriage was even right for her.

She found herself blaming her husband for the loss of her former self.

"Before dating Jack, I was good at making time for myself," she explained. "I went to weekly dance classes and worked on projects that excited me. I felt great! But everything changed this past year. I'm overwhelmed with responsibilities and constantly feel at the end of my rope. I can't even remember the last time I did anything just for me."

When Alice and Jack first started dating, she had invited him to join her for dance classes, but he declined. After a while, he began making offhand comments that left her feeling as though devoting time to classes was self-centered, especially when there were so many demands at work and at home. Eventually, Alice stopped dancing. She stopped making time for other hobbies too, like gardening and going on long walks in the morning. Before long, Alice started to burn out precisely because she had stopped doing those things that energized her. Now, she was exclusively pouring her energy into commitments that drained her.

This scenario is all too common among Generators. They set aside their passions and, unsurprisingly, their energy nosedives. I explained to Alice that, as a Generator, she had the most energy when she created space to engage with what she loved.

"It's crucial your husband understands and supports this need," I advised. This support might look like him lightening her responsibilities so she could do more of what she loved, asking questions about her passions, or even joining Alice in her favorite activities.

Alice realized Jack hadn't been providing any of this support. When Alice went home that evening, she explained to her husband that, despite their busy lives, she needed time for her passions—and that they were not superfluous. In fact, she told Jack reengaging with these activities on a regular basis would give her more energy to be fully present as a partner and mother.

Jack realized their relationship was on the line and that his approach was not inspiring Alice to show up as the best version of herself. He began taking the children on Saturday afternoons so she could attend dance classes, and they hired a babysitter once a month so he could join her. He made an effort to ask about her passions even though he didn't feel the need to discuss his own in the same way.

Over time, Alice began to remember that old, vibrant version of herself, and her frustration began to fall away. She realized that the distress she had been feeling wasn't about a fundamental flaw in her relationship with Jack but about her own unmet needs. Human Design offered her the language and permission to articulate those needs, which opened the door for change once she communicated them.

Practices

If you often find yourself frustrated, consider these practices as a way to move from discontent to satisfaction at work and in your relationships. And if you already feel fulfilled, these practices can help bring even more joy and contentment into your day-to-day life.

1. **Commit some of your energy to a hobby you love.**

   If you are dissatisfied with your career or responsibilities, you may find it helps to commit some of your energy to a favorite pastime, even if it's just an hour a week to start.

   Recommitting energy to something that is personally meaningful — whether it's attending a yoga class, dedicating an afternoon to photography, writing the novel you can't stop thinking about, or anything else that brings you joy — can remind you how it feels to be truly engaged and rekindle your natural enthusiasm. If you're unsure where to start, ask yourself: What would you feel glad to have done? Valuing your fulfillment is the first step toward tapping into your boundless energy and attracting better opportunities and relationships.

2. **Try preceding a mundane task with something that excites you.**

   Some mundane duties are inevitable, like taking out the trash or executing an annoying yet necessary task at work. One strategy to move through these obligations quickly and effectively is to precede the annoying task with one that excites you. For Generators, the energy gained from an energizing activity can often provide the momentum necessary to tackle the less satisfying ones.

   Mixing tasks you look forward to with those you're less enthusiastic about can help you balance your day. For instance, you might have a solo dance party before facing your taxes or wake up early to work on your website before addressing a work task you've been dreading. Put simply, leverage the energy gained from doing what you love to power through the essential tasks you don't enjoy.

3. **Consider whether you struggle to say *no* in any of your relationships.**

    Your energy is both finite and powerful, which makes it important to be discerning about where and how you use it. People may frequently seek your assistance because your vigor is so uplifting and bountiful. This is a beautiful thing . . . *but* you are only one person.

    Reflect on situations in which you agree to things you don't want to do or you feel unable to express when you don't have the energy to participate. Often, you might not have a specific reason; it simply doesn't feel right—and that's reason enough.

    If this pattern is present in your relationships, it might be time to assert your boundaries. Pay attention to how saying *no* and maintaining strong boundaries feels and consider having an open conversation with the other person about honoring your availability, even if that means not receiving the answer they hope to hear.

Journal Prompts

What parts of your life bring you the most joy, and why?

Do you love the work you do? If yes, why? If not, what's stopping you from going after work you love?

Do you set strong boundaries at work? If so, how does that feel? If not, what boundaries are important for you to establish, and why?

Do you feel like your relationships are equitable? If yes, what does balance in these relationships look like to you, and why? If not, how can you create more balance?

Do you expect the folks in your life to keep up with you? If yes, how's that working out? If no, how do you navigate the difference in pace?

KEY INSIGHTS

PERCENT OF POPULATION	30
TRADEMARK	Diversity
GIFTS	Being multipassionate, reinventing yourself, invigorating others with your enthusiasm, making things happen faster than anyone else, mastering new fields quickly, effortlessly pivoting between different projects
CHALLENGES	Feeling pressured to pick a lane, struggling to finish everything you start, lacking time or space to pursue your interests, experiencing boredom when confined to one task, staying with commitments for too long, taking on too much yourself, expecting others to match your pace
POPULAR ROLES	Investor, entrepreneur, executive, event producer, coach, speaker, musician, creative director, author, podcaster, artist, restaurateur (often balancing several of these simultaneously)
RELATIONSHIP NEEDS	Space to explore passions both together and independently, freedom to move at your pace, time to be in your own flow, flexibility to say yes or no without guilt, respect for your boundaries, no pressure to handle everything alone, freedom to change direction without judgment, support for your unconventional approach, curiosity about your current interests

Manifesting Generator

IN THE LATE 1990S, DWAYNE "THE ROCK" JOHNSON WAS AT THE PIN-
nacle of his wrestling career. His larger-than-life presence and multiple
championships made him one of World Wrestling Entertainment's biggest
stars. But that wasn't enough for The Rock.

In 1999, he made his acting debut on *That '70s Show* and within a few
years, became one of Hollywood's biggest action superheroes with films
like *The Mummy Returns*, the *Fast & Furious* franchise, and the Disney hit
Moana. Collectively, Johnson's films have grossed over $12.5 billion at
the box office, cementing his legacy as one of the biggest movie stars of
all time.

Since conquering Hollywood, Johnson has also founded a production company, a tequila brand, and even his own professional football
league.

"He's a freak of nature," said Jeffrey Dean Morgan, a friend and collaborator of Johnson's. "In the middle of shooting *Rampage*, he's off hosting
SNL and doing ads for Apple and running for president and whatever else.
He works out at 3:30 in the morning so he can get to set on time. I don't
know how he does it. And the other thing is, he's a family dude, so not only

is he juggling the nine million things he's got on his plate for work, he's also raising kids and got a happy marriage."

The Rock is a true Manifesting Generator in all his multipassionate, charismatic glory.

At Work

As a Manifesting Generator, your energy is limitless when you are genuinely excited about what you're doing, and you lift everyone around you with your electric presence.

Take my friend Natalia, for example. Natalia is like a human whirlwind, always moving, creating, and doing. One minute, she's brainstorming a new business idea; the next, she's writing her fourth book, and then she's off speaking to organizations and inspiring rooms with her story. Whenever I leave my time with her, I'm almost dizzy with excitement. In my experience, this is a hallmark of Manifesting Generators; they feel like the sun incarnate and always leave those around them buzzing with energy and inspiration.

As a Manifesting Generator, there is not a single box or role that can contain all of you—you are bigger than all of it. Manifesting Generators defy the belief that we must walk one single path to find fulfillment. You show us that success isn't about picking a lane; it's about welcoming continual evolution in our careers and lives. You thrive when you cultivate disparate and diverse career paths over the course of your life, or when you find a single role that satisfies your need for freshness and novelty, where each day feels different. One client shared that she excelled in her career only after becoming a freelancer. This meant every day offered something new, and she was free to set her own schedule as long as deadlines were met. Another shared, "I never used to know how to describe myself to people, so I would just pick one thing and compartmentalize my life. Now I don't have to. It's all me. Freedom."

You may struggle to adhere to conventional structures within a business or to follow an established route; this might feel limiting to your creative, dynamic nature. Many of my Manifesting Generator clients have discovered a traditional career is not the right long-term fit if it lacks flexibility and room for growth. You are at your best when each day offers new challenges and problems to solve. You can bounce your energy between different projects rather than feeling confined to just one. You are free to follow what invigorates you, even as it changes. You can master skills quickly and move on to the next just as fast. You don't feel guilty for changing direction, as you know it's a natural part of your process.

When you stay committed to tasks you no longer feel excited about based on a sense of pressure or obligation, you may struggle to tap into your naturally energetic nature and, instead, project sluggish, frustrated energy into the world. Or if your days are full of monotonous, repetitive tasks, you may become bored and burned out. Keeping your days fresh keeps your enthusiasm and excitement alive. As a fellow Manifesting Generator, Tina Turner once said, "If you are unhappy with anything . . . whatever is bringing you down, get rid of it. Because you'll find that when you're free, your true creativity, your true self, comes out."

It is also easy to burn out if you overextend yourself and say yes to commitments out of a desire to please, regardless of whether you actually have the time or energy, and then feel disappointed when you struggle to follow through. You only have the energy to make tasks happen with ease and speed when you are fulfilled by the endeavor or project at hand.

As a Manifesting Generator, you are naturally efficient and have a gift for finding the quickest way to make something happen, which might mean skipping some steps along the way. While speed is one of your gifts, it's not one everyone shares. I once had a Manifesting Generator client come to me after firing her seventh assistant. When I asked why, she said, "No one can keep up with my pace!" She was not disappointed by her assistant's competence but simply by their inability to move at her speed. I reminded her she might be better supported by those with complementary strengths rather than seeking someone just like her.

It's important that you lean into these differences as a Manifesting Generator because you may struggle if you skip steps and take shortcuts without having the right support. In an ideal world, you are surrounded by people who can handle the tasks you dislike so you can move quickly and skip steps without fear of dropping any balls. This will allow you to work at your natural speed while also ensuring everything runs smoothly. Generators or Projectors may be perfect collaborators for you, as Generators tend to love the step-by-step process of bringing ideas to life and Projectors are gifted at mastering systems that can make your life easier. It's also best to work with those who know you're designed to pivot quickly and are on board for it.

When evaluating career options, consider whether you'll have the freedom to work fast and maintain creative momentum, the opportunity to delegate or collaborate on tasks that drain your energy, a diversity of responsibilities, the level of autonomy you'll enjoy, and collaborators who understand and support your working style.

When you're on track at work, you'll feel a deep sense of satisfaction and peace at the end of the day. That feeling of being able to rest well once the day is over indicates you are energized by and connected to the work you are doing, and you've used up your energy doing work you love. (On the other hand, notice when you feel restless or unable to sleep—this indicates that your energy is not being put to use in the right direction.)

If you find yourself plagued with persistent frustration and anger, it may be because you are out of alignment in your career, and you're holding on to commitments you no longer have the energy for. This misalignment can look like a lack of inspiration or motivation to tackle challenges that arise, or an absence of freedom and flow in your days. Frustration invites you to consider whether a change is needed.

As a Manifesting Generator, free yourself from the idea that you must stick to one path, career, or project forever, and avoid any inclination to prioritize a career that makes sense to others over one that feels right to you intuitively. Each opportunity you are drawn to will serve a purpose and provide you with the tools and experience to master what comes next. As entrepreneur Michael Ventura puts it, "Not every project needs to live forever and doing what makes you feel good is more important than doing something that drains you." Always remember: your enthusiasm not only lights your path but also powers and lifts everyone around you.

The Renaissance Woman

When Susie logged in for our first session, it was as if my world suddenly became a bit brighter. This woman could light up a room with her enthusiasm—or in our case, a screen.

"Erin, I wish I'd met you twenty years ago!" she said in greeting.

Susie came to me because her cursory research into Human Design validated her impulses in a way no system had before, and she wanted to know more.

At sixty years old, Susie was a practicing lawyer, yet she knew she was destined for more than law alone. She had experimented with other passions over the years, such as dance and coaching but ultimately backed off for fear of doing too much or being misunderstood. Throughout her life, Susie had been led to believe that her lack of a singular focus was a bad thing, that if she could just "pick a lane," perhaps she would be more successful. "Susie, when will you decide what you want to be when you grow up?" her family often teased. Though lighthearted, their words made Susie doubt herself. But here's the thing: Susie and all Manifesting Generators are like Baby from *Dirty Dancing*—nobody puts them in a corner.

Still, Susie let her family's opinions influence her decisions for decades. She deferred her other passions to pursue law and forced herself to be methodical in her career choices rather than moving as fast or as freely as she wanted to.

Human Design confirmed what Susie had always known: her career path was not meant to be linear, and her passions were not meant to be singular. Only after discovering she was a Manifesting Generator did Susie finally give herself permission to see her multipassionate nature not as a flaw but as her greatest strength. She let go of the pressure to follow a traditional career path and instead embraced the pursuits that felt right, regardless of whether they made sense to others. She studied dance in the evenings and enrolled in a life-coaching certification. In a world that encourages specialization, Human Design allowed Susie to welcome the fact that she thrived in multiplicity.

Manifesting Generators move quickly, and Susie was no exception. Just six months after our session, she went part-time at her law firm, launched a life-coaching business, and began teaching dance classes in New York City. To the outside world, Susie's career might have looked scattered and unfocused. Yet to her, it finally felt perfect.

In Relationships

As a Manifesting Generator, your energy elevates those around you, making them feel more inspired, passionate, and excited about life.

However, your boundless and electric energy rests on your ability to build relationships in which you have the freedom to say yes or no to commitments without feeling guilty or facing judgment from others. If others see your natural capacity as a reason to burden you with all the responsibilities, you may become overwhelmed and drained. This affects not only you but also those around you, who will be able to sense your exhaustion and burden.

One of your most essential needs in relationships is the space to pursue what genuinely excites you, both with others and on your own. While it's wonderful to engage in shared passions with friends, the reality is that no one can match your pace all the time. I've seen couples that include a Manifesting Generator thrive by indulging their separate interests during the day and reconnecting in the evening, when both are recharged by their individual pursuits. The opposite is also true. I've counseled many clients whose Manifesting Generator partner, when frustrated and unhappy with their job, brings that same lethargy into their home life, causing their discontent to permeate the family.

It may initially feel revolutionary to prioritize your joy and desires in your relationships, especially if you've spent much of your life living in a more sacrificial way, tending to everyone else's needs above your own. Yet following your excitement is what allows you to show up as your brightest self in your relationships. In an ideal world, those close to you understand the importance of allowing you the space to pursue what you love and know that your ability to get things done doesn't mean you should carry all the responsibilities alone. They care about what you genuinely have the energy for and actively lessen your load so that you have more room to engage in what excites you. Of course, you participate in shared responsibilities, but time to pursue what naturally energizes you is seen as necessary, not selfish.

While it may not be possible all the time, explore whether you can set aside specific times—maybe a morning, an afternoon, or even a day each week—when you can immerse yourself in your interests without guilt or interruption. One of my Manifesting Generator clients built a shed in his backyard as a retreat where he could step away from family once a day to engage in woodworking. This personal time to dive into his own projects allowed him to return to his family rejuvenated and more present. As with Generators, it's especially important as a Manifesting Generator parent that you carve out time for what naturally revitalizes you, even if it doesn't involve your kids. This boosts your energy and inspires you to show up as a vibrant force at home. It can also be useful to consider the activities that feel particularly fun to dive into with your kids and to prioritize those.

It's crucial for Manifesting Generators to allow partners their own space as well, regardless of their Type. As a Manifesting Generator, your energy is expansive and powerful—while it can inspire, it can also overwhelm, especially when others feel pressured to keep up. Giving your partner room to connect with themselves is essential too.

One of the most significant realizations among my Manifesting Generator clients is that not everyone can move as quickly or multitask as effectively. One client explained, "Expecting my Generator husband to keep up with my style, which is juggling a thousand projects at once, is unrealistic and sets us up for failure." Manifesting Generators are often disappointed with the comparatively low capacity of others until they understand that their own ability to move quickly, balance multiple projects, and pivot effortlessly is a unique gift, not a universal trait.

As a Manifesting Generator, you might feel misunderstood in relationships if your need for a diversity of activities, work, and hobbies is misinterpreted as a lack of focus. For instance, your passions for poetry, coding, and modeling might read as indecisive, when it simply means you have range. You may feel constrained if others try to categorize you in ways that are easy for them to understand but that don't naturally fit you. It's not necessary for others to fully understand everything you do. What *is* important is that those close to you accept your multidimensionality without making you feel scattered or misguided, trusting that if it feels right to you, it's right.

For Manifesting Generators, an ideal relationship allows for constant evolution, whether through major life changes or daily decisions, like committing to dinner one week prior and backing out the day of when the energy for it is no longer there. It's important to establish that you thrive on change so your relationships can support your dynamic energy. It's not about you being flaky or fickle; it's about embracing your innate need for flexibility and committing to what feels right, while allowing room to adjust as necessary. The right people will understand they get the best of you when you show up to commitments with a full-bodied yes. As one Manifesting Generator client put it, "My close friends know better than to make fixed plans with me. My usual response is, 'I'll see how I feel that day.' Their understanding removes the pressure to commit too early or for the wrong reasons." Another said, "I now give a tentative yes or no, but also make it clear I might change my mind. This flexibility is incredibly liberating." It is helpful to learn to balance your need for spontaneity with others' potential preference for predictability and routine so that both of your needs are respected.

Because your interests continually evolve, it's important to be in relationships with people who are curious about what excites and energizes you currently rather than being questioned about the shifts you are making or encouraged to pick things back up from the past. They want to know what's bringing you life right now. You should feel no shame that what you were interested in at the last family gathering is not what you're interested in at the next.

While some relationships may be obligatory, make sure to create ample space for those that bring deep satisfaction and fulfillment rather than continual frustration. Just as you are meant to be energized by your work, you should be lifted by your relationships and spend the majority of your time with those who give you more energy than they take.

Many Gifts

Sahara sought me out because she was struggling in her relationship with her father, who also happened to be one of the most important forces in her life. Their disconnect was wrecking Sahara. She began to cry almost as soon as we sat down in a cozy corner of an outdoor café.

Sahara had just turned thirty and loved her eclectic life even though she knew it didn't always make sense to others, especially those she'd grown up with. Over the past decade, she had lived in five cities, completed a yoga teacher certification, opened a juice shop, and worked as a freelance copywriter. Just recently, she had embarked on a master's program in fiction writing. She was never bored, and each new adventure tapped into a part of herself that felt unexplored.

Yet Sahara's father saw her career as haphazard. Having been a physician for forty years, he valued hard work toward a singular goal. He expected Sahara to follow a similar trajectory and was frustrated with what he perceived as her lack of direction. Sahara felt ashamed that she wasn't meeting her father's expectations. But she was also confused. Sahara found her career to be varied, rich, and purposeful.

Sahara breathed a huge sigh of relief upon learning that her multipassionate, nonlinear path was a natural expression of her personality as a Manifesting Generator.

"I've been internalizing my father's disappointment," she said, beginning to lighten up a little. "It's such a relief to learn I'm fine just as I am."

By urging her to emulate his own style of ambition, Sahara's father inadvertently made her feel insecure about her innate multihyphenate ability. Of *course* they felt disconnected.

Human Design gave Sahara the framework she needed to confront her father and explain that her choices stemmed from authenticity, not a lack of dedication. Over the course of many conversations, including one I participated in, her father began to understand that his frustration came not from the fact that something was wrong with Sahara but from expecting her to be just like him.

In the months that followed, Sahara and her father grew closer than ever. For the first time in years, she felt inspired to share what she was working on with him, and he learned to ask questions without judgment. He even started reading the fiction she wrote in her master's program and attending her yoga classes. Along the way, he discovered that, although Sahara's path wasn't traditional, what she possessed was powerful—not just one gift, but *many*.

Practices

If you feel weighed down by frustration or anger, consider these practices as ways to bring more satisfaction, peace, and freedom into your work and relationships. Even if you are already feeling enthusiastic and fulfilled, they can ensure you stay right on track.

1. **Give yourself permission to pivot, regardless of what others think.**

    It's natural for you to try things on and then move on; this is a key part of how you work. If you're unsure if a job or commitment is right for you, consider whether you're sticking with it just because you or others think you should. It may have once been a fit but no longer is, or perhaps it was never a fit to begin with.

Letting go can be hard, especially when you fear disappointing others, but remember this: *no one benefits from your halfhearted yes.* Moving on from what no longer inspires you makes room for the things that do. Your energy comes alive when you are wholehearted about what you're working on. Glennon Doyle put it perfectly when she wrote in *Untamed*, "Every time you're given a choice between disappointing someone else and disappointing yourself, your duty is to disappoint that someone else." When you honor your changing desires, you'll feel better, and others will enjoy being around you more—it's a natural result of doing what you love.

It may be useful to have conversations with those close to you—like partners, collaborators, or friends—about your need to keep things fresh. This can help them understand and respect your needs instead of seeing them as negative because they differ from their own. And if they don't get it . . . well, that's okay too. What matters most is that you remain true to yourself and spread that beautiful, contagious excitement of yours to all who are lucky enough to cross your path.

2. **Practice delegating the step-by-step tasks that drain you.**

You shine brightest when you can move quickly, bypass steps, and stay in your creative flow. Often, this will require that you delegate tedious pieces that feel mundane to you but are exciting to someone else. Never forget that what seems dull to you could be someone else's dream. As a first step, simply write down the steps that you would hand off to someone else in an ideal world.

Whether it's at home or work, consider asking for help and letting go of the idea that you must handle everything yourself. The more you free your energy from activities that drain you, the more energy you have to dedicate to activities that enliven you, and the more everyone around you benefits from that increased energy flow.

3. **Set aside time to be in your own uninterrupted flow.**

To release the expectation that others match your speed and to honor your natural need for independence, carve out a block of time on at least a weekly basis to dive into activities you love, free from disruptions.

Whether it's a mini writers' retreat, a Human Design class, building a LEGO set you've been dreaming of, making music, or gardening, dedicate this time to something that brings you joy and that you're doing simply because you want to. After you've spent this time in your own flow, reflect on how you feel. Are you more revitalized and energetic? Do you find that taking this time not only enriches you but also positively impacts everyone you spend time with?

Journal Prompts

What is currently bringing you the most satisfaction in your life, and why?

Do you feel pressure to stick to a linear path in your career? If so, how does that feel? If not, what approach feels more natural, and why?

Are there any projects you're holding on to that you no longer have the energy for? If so, how's that working out?

Do you often find yourself disappointed with the pace of others? If yes, how is that impacting your relationships? How would it feel to recognize that not everyone moves at your speed?

Which relationships allow you to grow and change rather than hold you to a static version of yourself? How do those relationships make you feel, and why?

KEY INSIGHTS

PERCENT OF POPULATION	23
TRADEMARK	Perspective
GIFTS	Seeing the big picture, mastering systems, spotting patterns, improving efficiency, recognizing potential in others, making people feel seen, asking insightful questions, leading
CHALLENGES	Burning out from working too hard on the wrong things, feeling ashamed for needing rest, not knowing when to stop, tying your worth to how much you do, absorbing others' frustration and feeling drained, feeling unseen and underappreciated
POPULAR ROLES	Coach, advisor, leader, teacher, manager, researcher, author, podcaster, therapist, counselor, consultant, founder, artist, agent, investor, lawyer
RELATIONSHIP NEEDS	Space for alone time and rest, respect for your point of view, appreciation for your contributions, consideration of your energy levels, quality one-on-one time, deep connection, support, awareness of your sensitivity to others' energy

Projector

ONE DAY IN 1994, WHILE CAMPAIGNING FOR THE PRESIDENCY OF South Africa, Nelson Mandela and the coauthor of his autobiography, Richard Stengel, boarded a small plane to Natal, formerly a province in South Africa, where Mandela was scheduled to give a speech to his supporters. Midflight, Mandela glanced out the window and noticed that one of the propellers had stopped turning. Without a trace of alarm, he turned to Stengel and said, "You might want to inform the pilot that the propeller isn't working." Then, he casually returned to his newspaper.

In an interview with PBS, Stengel recalled feeling terrified with the possibility of death looming large. The only way he managed to stay composed was by keeping his eyes on Mandela, who remained calm throughout the ordeal. In his book *Mandela's Way*, Stengel reflected that Mandela was the kind of leader people looked to for courage and strength, and that "Even when the weight of the world was on his shoulders, he would wear it lightly."

That same year, Nelson Mandela became the first democratically elected president of South Africa and shepherded a nation torn apart by apartheid and war into a new era of reconciliation and peace. As a consummate leader and guide known for his subtlety and wisdom, Nelson Mandela was a Projector.

How Do You Choose?

At Work

As a Projector, you are naturally insightful and intuitive. You can easily sense people's potential and how they can leverage their gifts to work more effectively. Your ability to read a room, person, or situation makes you the team member everyone wants in important meetings because your perspective is invaluable. You might find teammates and clients turn to you in challenging moments because they trust your advice and guidance. You can see to the heart of the matter and observe where things could be done differently in ways others miss. Your true gifts lie in your bird's-eye view and deep attunement to others, not in how hard you work or how much you achieve.

The most natural position for you is as a leader or guide, where you can rise above it all, ask the right questions, and offer your perspective on what's happening. In a role purely focused on execution, you can quickly burn out and feel unable to access and tap into these gifts.

As a Projector, you also have a gift for building and understanding systems. This could look like devising a system to support others or refining an existing process to make it more efficient. Or it might mean mastering a system or modality, becoming an expert, and sharing your perspective on it with the world.

How well you manage your energy directly affects your ability to tap into these gifts. Your energy fluctuates throughout the day, and following your natural rhythm—leveraging your energy when it's high and taking rest when it's low—is the pathway to heightened creativity, inspiration, and efficacy. You live in a world of doers, but that doesn't mean you have to be one too. If you try to keep up with the world around you, you can easily wear yourself out. Whereas the more you allow yourself to rest, the easier it is to connect to your gifts. An artist client found that trying to keep pace with her collaborators stifled her creativity, but when she was rested, her creativity bloomed. An entrepreneur added flow days to her calendar, days during which she booked nothing at all, and became far more productive and inspired. Space allowed for inspiration, while a packed schedule did not.

One of my NBA clients managed his demanding career by making rest a priority, often heading home early while his teammates stayed out. Another client burned out working a nine-to-five job. Upon learning that she wasn't meant to be "on" all the time, she transitioned into self-employment and entered the coaching industry, finding it more flexible and ultimately more successful for her. While long breaks might not be feasible in your line of work, even a five-minute tea or bathroom break can rejuvenate you and make a difference.

As tempting as it can be to overexert yourself and try to do it all, it's important to learn to accept help as a Projector, especially the kind that allows your strengths to shine. You may find you work well with Generators or Manifesting Generators, who provide the juice to consistently make things happen; this allows you to honor your natural rhythms and step into your role as leader, guide, or teacher.

Understanding this has been liberating for me as a Projector. I still fall into the trap of overworking, only to be reminded time and time again that doing more doesn't make me better or more effective. My husband recognizes this too. When he sees me working late, he'll gently ask, "Why are you still at it?" I usually realize there's no good reason, so I take that as an invitation to shut down for the day. Human Design has shown me that my strength lies in seeing, not doing, and my gifts come alive when I'm well-rested, not when I'm pushing myself too hard. As author and professor Cal Newport reminds us in *Slow Productivity*, "This is what ultimately matters: where you end up, not the speed at which you get there, or the number of people you impress with your jittery busyness along the way."

As a Projector, you're particularly attuned to the creative energy of others and their feelings about their work. When you work around those energized by what they're working on (particularly enthusiastic Generators or Manifesting Generators), their energy rubs off on you, and you may find more energy to make things happen. On the other hand, if you work around people who are frustrated and depleted, their sluggishness can also rub off on you, leaving you to feel exhausted. You may be the first to notice when someone is nearing burnout. Consider who feels energetically healthy and energizing to be around; these are the right collaborators for you. Also, be mindful that being around those who are constantly doing might pressure you to keep up and do more, even when it's not natural for you. Be conscious of when it's time to step away from others' constant energy and reconnect with yourself.

An ideal career offers a flexible schedule that allows you to honor the ebbs and flows of your energy and take breaks when needed. Your collaborators do not expect you to be available all the time and understand that you are most effective when rested and inspired. Your schedule is not booked back-to-back and includes built-in space and rest. You balance output and creation with ample time for input, continually learning and refining your expertise. You have the opportunity to leverage your big-picture perspective and skill for understanding people. Your talents and insights are valued above your ability to put in continuous effort. You can delegate tasks and receive support. The environment nurtures your growth into leadership or a role where you can fully focus on your craft.

As a Projector, you are meant to achieve success on your own terms. This can look like success rooted in ease, space, and support, rather than hustle and burnout, and success that feels as good as it looks. Success likely feels as if you are valued and compensated for your distinct talents and perspective. This kind of appreciation energizes you and signals you're on the right path.

You may start to feel bitter in a scenario where you feel out of alignment with your work. This bitterness is often rooted in feeling unseen or uninvited to share your gifts or perspective. Maybe you see how processes can be improved in the team or environment around you, yet no one is asking for your insights. Or perhaps everyone asks for your advice, but they don't act on it, nor do they compensate you for it. Or maybe you're trying to keep up with a pace that isn't sustainable and burning yourself out in the process. Persistent bitterness offers you an opportunity to check in with yourself and assess whether or not an opportunity or situation is still correct for you.

The key to tapping into your gifts as a Projector is to begin to trust the natural cycles of your energy rather than expecting yourself to produce all the time. Watch your gifts come alive when you step off the constant productivity treadmill that so many of us have become lost in, and allow rest to create space for inspiration to flow back into your life.

From Burnout to Balance

When I began working at a start-up fresh out of college, I was full of energy and eager to dive in. The team welcomed my enthusiasm, and I quickly became the go-to person for advice, support, and guidance—a role I genuinely enjoyed. It was the same role I had played in every space I found myself in, personal or professional. But all this was in addition to my *actual* role at the start-up, which meant I had to find time to answer customer support emails, devise marketing strategies, and handle operations. Before long, not only was I the first to arrive at the office every day but I was also pulling all-nighters. I began to realize that my pace was unsustainable. I simply couldn't maintain the excitement I had begun with.

Rather than recognizing that being constantly "on" was burning me out, I believed my exhaustion meant something was wrong with me. I felt that my worth hinged on constant productivity and that tireless effort was the key to achievement.

After a while, I started to wonder if I just wasn't cut out for success. I also began to resent that I wasn't being paid or recognized for what felt like my true talents: asking good questions, offering helpful insights, and making people feel seen. And yet the idea that a job could center around these strengths or that I could find success in a way that felt sustainable seemed almost impossible.

It wasn't until I discovered I was a Projector that I realized my curiosity and people skills were talents big enough to build a career around. I also (finally) understood that hustling, while frequently tempting and sometimes appropriate, would more often guarantee burnout than success. Once I embraced this about myself, my life began to change in meaningful ways: I stopped equating relentless activity with achievement, acknowledged that always being available wasn't a measure of accomplishment, recognized that my energy ebbed and flowed just as nature does, and accepted that my gifts were more about making people feel seen than making things happen.

I know I'm not alone in this. So often, we obsess about how a career looks, valuing appearance over the genuine experience of how it feels. For me, it wasn't until my career *felt* right—in other words, balanced and aligned with my unique gifts—that I finally experienced the success and impact I'd always dreamed of.

In Relationships

Your capacity to make people feel seen and understood naturally draws them to you, making you a friend magnet. It's important to be selective in your relationships and invest in people who desire the depth of connection you offer. Build relationships with those who do not shy away from intensity, appreciate your deep-feeling nature, and are comfortable being seen by you. One client shared she had been made fun of throughout her life for asking deep questions off the bat. Over time, she came to realize this was not a personal flaw but simply an indication that certain people weren't right for her. Another client shared how small talk or surface-level conversations were an immediate turnoff because she needed to be able to ask thought-provoking questions and have them engaged with.

However, deeply understanding others without feeling seen or appreciated in return can leave you feeling exhausted and taken advantage of. Reciprocity in your relationships is essential. One client felt like she was always working, even in friendships, because people constantly sought her wisdom but rarely acknowledged her efforts or showed interest in knowing her beyond the advice she gave. Another client shared that a friend frequently asked for guidance but never acted on any of it, which left her feeling unrecognized and drained from giving so much with little in return. To gauge reciprocity, consider who asks thoughtful questions, listens, and shows a genuine interest in understanding how you operate and see the world. You shouldn't always have to be the one asking questions or initiating conversations, a role that you easily fall into because you're naturally good at it. The effort should go both ways. You, too, deserve to be invited to take up space in someone's world and asked questions in a way that makes you feel as if the other person sees you and wants to know even more. This doesn't mean you should feel pressure to share, but you *should* sense sincere curiosity from the person you're interacting with.

As a Projector myself, I can attest to the fact that my social circle transformed once I understood my need for reciprocity. I've always been good at empathizing with others and had many friends because of it, but until I understood the importance not just of giving but also receiving, I rarely felt seen myself. Once I started prioritizing reciprocity, the number of friends in my life diminished, but those who remained—and came into my life from that point forward—became much more meaningful. It's likely quality will trump quantity in your relationships too. You may find more fulfillment in having a few close, meaningful relationships rather than a big circle of acquaintances and prioritizing one-on-one time with those who make you feel most understood. One-on-one time is a natural setting for you to see others and feel recognized in return. One client described feeling disconnected in his relationships and noted how that coincided with a lack of one-on-one time with his children and closest friends. When he made spending time with each person individually a priority, the depth of his connections returned. As a Projector, it's important to take the time to consider the gatherings and social engagements that fill your cup.

One of my Projector clients, whose partner is a Manifesting Generator, found that learning their distinct designs helped her understand why they showed up to social occasions so differently. While her partner loved bouncing around and meeting new people, she preferred deep, intimate conversations in a quiet corner. This understanding helped them appreciate their differences and refrain from imposing unrealistic expectations on each other when they went out together.

How Do You Choose?

Projectors often feel deeply sensitive to others' energy and may require more time to recharge and rest in relationships as a result. It may feel counterintuitive to distance yourself from loved ones, but taking time just for you is one of the simplest and most effective ways to unwind and return to your center. This could mean attending an exercise class by yourself, spending an evening journaling, enjoying a slow morning alone, lying on the bathroom floor for a few minutes of solitude, sleeping alone some nights, dining out solo, or even taking a trip by yourself. It's important that your people respect—and even encourage—your need for replenishment and self-care. You should feel free and comfortable to rest regularly without concern that resentment will build up in your relationship as a result. Others also shouldn't expect you to always be available for a conversation, even if you're in a shared space.

As a Projector parent, it is especially important that you find time for yourself to pause and restore, even if it's just stepping away for a moment. One mother shared that before she understood her Type, she used to think she was a bad mom simply because she found her child's energy overwhelming at times and needed some space. Learning she was a Projector released the guilt she'd long been carrying.

Another client shared that learning her husband is a Projector means she no longer gets annoyed when he lies down to rest in the middle of the day even when there are tasks that need to be done. In fact, she now *encourages* it, knowing he'll be more present and engaged afterward. Another Projector client likened herself to a cat, recognizing her need to occasionally do nothing and rest. When she finds herself overwhelmed and burned out, her partner is now often the first to ask her: "Have you taken the time to be a cat today?" It's important to feel acknowledged for your presence and the natural shift you inspire in a room instead of only feeling valued for the number of chores you complete or how much you can accomplish in a day.

Unlike some who can work right up until bedtime, you benefit from winding down before you feel tired. This might mean a bedtime routine that differs from a partner's, such as getting into bed early to read or journal, perhaps even in your own space. I am married to a Generator, and we've always had our own bedrooms. I cherish getting into bed by 8:30 p.m. to unwind with a novel, while he often works on the things he's passionate about long after I've called it a day. For us, separate bedrooms aren't about always sleeping apart but about honoring our distinct rhythms and the ability to choose when to share the same space rather than having it be the default.

As a Projector, you operate differently from most, which means it's critical to be clear about what you need to thrive in connection. Others may not intuitively or easily grasp how you operate. Communicating your needs might mean explaining to friends and family that your energy levels fluctuate daily. You might not always have the stamina to keep up with them or stay out late; rest may be a higher priority for you. Instead of expecting consistent participation from you, they can check in to see what you're up for at any given moment and recognize your constant presence isn't the only measure of your friendship. It might mean telling your family you need to take a break from a big gathering or letting a partner know you need regular alone time or even prefer sleeping separately.

The right relationships are those that leave you feeling successful, seen, and valued; unsustainable ones might leave you feeling bitter and underappreciated. Pay attention to these feelings, because they will guide you toward the most fulfilling relationships.

From Self-Doubt to Self-Trust

Joanna never quite felt like enough in her partnership. Her husband, Andrew, is a go-getter whom people admire for his ability to manage multiple businesses, be an active father to four children, and run marathons on the side. Joanna was inspired by him too. But she struggled to keep pace and wondered if something was fundamentally wrong with her.

As she shared her story, Joanna hunched over, almost folding in on herself. It was clear how conflicted she felt: her deep love for Andrew was clouded by self-doubt, and she was even starting to question the future of their relationship simply because she couldn't match his stamina.

"I am so proud of everything he's achieved," she told me, "but there's a part of me that feels inadequate. Andrew is relentless! He always wants to be on the move, even on weekends, whereas I need breaks and time to myself. He isn't satisfied unless he's creating something new, while I cherish the moments of stillness in my career and life. Sometimes, he doesn't understand why I can't keep up. Does this mean we're just not a match?"

I explained to Joanna that, according to their designs, she and her husband were indeed opposites. Andrew, a quintessential Manifesting Generator, wakes up with a full tank each day and needs to exhaust that energy in order to feel fulfilled. In contrast, Joanna's Projector energy ebbs and flows. She requires regular rest and solitude, *especially* because she lives with such a dynamic partner.

As a Projector myself, I could practically feel Joanna's exhale as I assured her that nothing was wrong with her. At the end of our session, Joanna expressed gratitude that she was able to gain a greater appreciation for her husband's drive while also feeling more compassionate toward herself.

The next week, Joanna and I met again—this time with her husband. It turned out to be one of the most powerful conversations I've witnessed in a decade of practice. It became clear that, although Joanna didn't possess Andrew's tirelessness, her contributions were invaluable. She might not have the energy to play outside with her kids for hours or to show up for each and every activity, but she served as the family's lodestar, making them feel understood and serving as a confidante and counselor in times of need. While Joanna wasn't out there building companies, her behind-the-scenes guidance was crucial. Andrew admitted that much of his success could be attributed to her wisdom about which direction to take.

> Joanna was moved to tears as Andrew acknowledged her vital role and recognized the unrealistic expectations he had placed on her. Human Design gave them permission to embrace their individual approaches and celebrate how essential each was to creating a balanced home.

Practices

If you often find yourself feeling bitter or underappreciated, consider these practices as ways to help you find more success and respect in your work and relationships. And if you already feel successful, these practices can support you in discovering new levels of recognition.

1. **Pay attention to any modalities or systems you feel drawn to learn.**

   Rather than seeing studying as just a hobby or an unnecessary or unproductive use of your time, consider it a pathway to uncovering your next steps. You have a knack for mastering, teaching, and creating systems—and you also might just simply love learning. Start noticing whether you feel drawn to learning or sharing any modalities or systems, especially those that offer deeper insights into understanding and guiding people.

   Embracing your natural curiosity is a beautiful way to move beyond any tendencies you have to measure your worth by how much you do and instead, connect with the unique gifts you're meant to share with the world.

2. **Build in moments of pause and rest in your days.**

   You might feel compelled to keep working or doing simply because you think you should, but this often leads to diminishing returns. Doing more does not make you more effective, but regular rest and space do.

Try something different. Build in small moments of pause throughout the day, during which you release the need to be productive. Instead, allow yourself to just be. Take a short walk, sit with a cup of tea, take a nap, or read your favorite book for twenty minutes. When you integrate breaks into your days, how do you feel? What do you notice about the quality of your work and life?

3. **Prioritize one-on-one quality time with people who make you feel seen.**

My friendships deepened when I realized large group gatherings weren't always fulfilling for me and I made more intimate one-on-one time to connect with friends a priority. I scheduled regular calls with my friends who lived across the country, reached out to my favorite friends for time to connect one-on-one (even if we'd just had dinner with our partners the week before), and made it a practice to call friends when I was driving.

Whether they're your friends, partners, family members, colleagues, or children, take the time to consider which relationships bring you the most fulfillment, recognition, and depth, and make it a point to prioritize one-on-one time with these people in whatever way feels sustainable and feasible for you. Notice how deepening these individual connections shifts your feeling of success and contentment in these relationships and your social world.

Journal Prompts

What parts of your life make you feel the most successful, and why?

Where is your perspective valued over your ability to produce? How does that feel, and do you want more of it?

Do you take breaks during the day? If so, how do they impact your productivity and happiness? If not, why?

Who meets you at the level of depth you desire? How does that feel, and would you like to experience that more often?

Which social environments are the most fulfilling for you, and why?

KEY INSIGHTS

PERCENT OF POPULATION	10
TRADEMARK	Boldness
GIFTS	Getting new ideas off the ground, being unabashedly unafraid to live a life that feels authentic to you, forging your own path, being the first, challenging norms, transforming the way things are done, igniting a fire under others, showing up in a way that inspires and provokes
CHALLENGES	Getting bogged down in the day-to-day minutia of keeping new ideas running in the long run, trying to complete everything you start, struggling to fit into a conventional role, playing it small, working without rest
POPULAR ROLES	Entrepreneur, artist, innovator, thought leader, inventor, consultant, creative director, freelancer, speaker, activist, performer
RELATIONSHIP NEEDS	Independence, freedom to do things your way, appreciation of your need for solitude, depth without feeling smothered, respect for your energy cycles, space to share your visions, reminders of your impact, support, a secure connection, love for your adventurous spirit

Manifestor

IN 1944 MAYA ANGELOU HAD A DREAM—TO BECOME A STREETCAR conductor in her hometown of San Francisco. In her book *Mom & Me & Mom*, she recalled how much she loved their uniforms: "I had seen women on the streetcars with their little moneychanging belts and with bibs on their caps and well-fitted uniforms." She had watched many people wear those uniforms, but none of them were Black women, and she was determined to be the first.

So, at fifteen years old, she took a year off of high school and applied for a position. At first, they rejected her. But as she describes in her famous work *I Know Why the Caged Bird Sings*, she returned every day for two weeks until they finally allowed her to put in an application. She got the job.

It would be the first of many glass ceilings to shatter in the wake of Angelou's unbridled ambitions. Eventually, she became Hollywood's first Black woman director, the first Black woman to write a screenplay for a major movie, the first Black woman on a US coin, and the first woman to deliver an inaugural poem in US history.

Maya Angelou was a poet, storyteller, activist, artist, educator, pioneer, and, fittingly, a Manifestor.

How Do You Choose?

At Work

As a Manifestor, you are a natural disruptor and trailblazer. You shake up any space or team you enter and bring new ideas, movements, and ways of doing things into the world, igniting the spark that others follow and rally around. Like Maya Angelou, who broke new ground and paved the way for countless others, you are meant to be the first. You are often ahead of the curve, seeing how the tide is changing long before others do, whether it's in people, teams, communities, or societies. When embraced, this gift can revolutionize and transform but, if misunderstood, your energy and insights might be perceived as threatening or challenging to the status quo.

I've had many Manifestor clients struggle in corporate environments where they could easily see what was coming down the line and where innovation was needed, yet no one wanted to listen. The truth they saw would require change the leaders did not want. This kind of environment is deeply draining—and even distressing—to Manifestors. To avoid this, seek collaborators and creative partners who celebrate your disruptive nature and foresight. You're at your best when you feel free to innovate and challenge conventional methods and aren't expected to execute in the same old familiar way.

One therapist shared with me, "I started at a group practice but felt shut down and controlled by the owner when I voiced my ideas. Now, I run my own practice because I've learned I cannot be told how to do things." Another client took over an existing business and, at first, tried to maintain the status quo. Not only did it feel awful, it didn't work. Only when she allowed herself to change everything from the ground up did the business start to succeed.

As a Manifestor, your gift is jumpstarting new ideas, not maintaining old ones. You excel at lighting a fire under others, inspiring them to move forward in a different direction. You might struggle if you try to handle everything at work—the initiating and the sustaining—rather than focusing on your talent for getting things started, or if you commit to long-term projects that don't acknowledge that your energy often peaks at the project's outset. You can and should delegate so that you can free up your energy to initiate and breathe life into new projects. This is where your strength lies. You may pair well with those who can sustain the ideas you envision, like Generators, or those who can guide and manage a team to execute your visions, like Projectors.

Day to day, it is important to experience a sense of freedom and control, and to have the opportunity to make tasks happen on your own terms. Being expected to operate within a team all the time or having little space to work independently can feel constraining. In an optimal situation, you have the autonomy to stay in your creative flow on a regular basis, act on fresh impulses and ideas, and make decisions without constant oversight or approval. My Manifestor clients have often found the most success when they're self-employed or in a team setting that affords them flexibility and freedom within their clear area of responsibility. For instance, one client thrived in a corporate role where his primary task was to seek out new partnerships. He flourished because he and his boss agreed on the goal but left the approach up to him.

One reason flexibility is optimal is that your energy comes in creative bursts. Like Projectors, you are not meant to take action consistently. The difference is that your energy may not ebb and flow on a daily basis like it does for Projectors. Rather, you are driven by inspiration, and may find that you can make a lot happen in a surge of inspiration over a couple of hours, days, or weeks. Once the inspiration has been tethered, this burst of energy may be followed by a period in which you need to rest and be alone, whether it's for hours, days, or weeks. This might mean disappearing every so often to recharge alone and await your next burst of inspiration. It's important that your collaborators understand the need to give you the space for your inspiration to come alive, and do not expect you to be "on" and available all the time. In an ideal world, your work schedule is flexible, respects your natural cycles, and offers solitude and downtime when you need it. If that is not possible in your current role, find small ways to incorporate solitude and rest into your days—like spending a night alone after a long day of work or choosing a quieter, more private spot in the office when your energy is low.

A sense of peace will let you know that you're on the right track in your career. This can look like experiencing minimal resistance or restriction from others, and having the space and support necessary to dream up and pursue your visions. You do what you want when you want. You feel empowered, in control, and free. You see the depth of your impact.

Whereas if you often feel angry, it's a signal that something in your career needs to change. Anger can arise when you lack autonomy and control over your work and schedule. When others dictate what you do and how you do it, it can feel as if the world is pushing against you, preventing you from realizing your ideas. If you're burdened with making everything happen and can't honor that your energy is strongest at the start of a project, you may become resentful and exhausted. Anger flags the fact that you need to check in with yourself, assess whether an opportunity or approach is still right, and make adjustments if necessary.

So often, I've sat with Manifestors who have been afraid to step into their power in their careers for fear of being too big or rocking the boat, their spirit dampened by teams that found their provocative, initiating nature threatening in the past. *Manifestors, I want you to remember this: your daring, inciting nature is your gift.* You are here to spark the changes the world around you needs and to boldly tread your own path. As Maya Angelou once said, "If you're always trying to be normal, you will never know how amazing you can be."

The Fire Starter

Even before George and I met, I could feel his intensity through our email exchanges. He was full of conviction, yet I could also sense a creeping feeling of defeat.

George was a serial entrepreneur with zero wins to his name—so far. He had started a lot of companies but struggled to keep any of them afloat long enough to see success. He came to me wondering if he might be better off as a rank-and-file employee at an established organization instead of consistently taking swings as an entrepreneur.

"I hit the same wall every time," he explained. "The beginning is exhilarating, but I can't keep the momentum going. Maybe I'm not cut out for this."

I could feel a surge of excitement when he spoke about launching something new, and watched the spark dim whenever the conversation turned to maintaining what he had begun.

"George," I said, smiling, "your instinct is right on. Giving birth to new ideas is your sweet spot; sustaining them is *not*." I watched as he let out a relieved sigh.

It's easy to understand why hearing this was a comfort to George. He had regularly felt like a failure for running out of energy when it came to seeing through what he started. Once he let go of the shame associated with perceived failure and realized his gifts lay in initiating, he was able to focus his efforts on building a team of collaborators who could take over after his initial burst of energy set his vision into motion.

The last time we checked in, George was beaming, and that underlying sense of defeat had vanished. His latest venture was thriving under the management of his team, and he was already onto the next big idea.

"I light the fire," he said, "and they keep it burning."

George felt free and his energy was larger than life. This was a huge transformation from the weighed-down man I had met just a few months earlier. George's career transformed when he stepped into his calling as a starter and learned when to step back and hand the reins to others.

In Relationships

Years ago, my Human Design side hustle was taking off, but I was still working full-time at a company I loved. I knew it was time to leave the company, but I hadn't yet convinced myself to take the leap. As I was mulling over this on my way to meet with my boss, I happened to run into my Manifestor friend. She looked at me and said, "Erin, it's time. This is your moment. Let him know you're stepping away to build your business."

As soon as she suggested it, I knew I must. Heeding her advice, I walked into my boss's office and shared that it was time for me to go all in on my business.

My experience with Manifestors is often like this. They have an uncanny ability to effortlessly guide others toward their next big experience in life. They usually don't even realize how impactful and initiatory their presence can be. It is not that they are necessarily loud or overbearing; they just have a natural intensity that commands attention. When they walk into a room, you can feel the energy shift.

As a Manifestor, you are a breath of fresh air in relationships because you possess naturally provocative, inspiring, and expansive energy. That's why it's important to be in relationships that offer the space for you to express yourself fully and boldly. You may struggle if you choose relationships that disconnect you from your innate power and make you feel small, or if others perceive your power as threatening and something to be controlled. This is especially problematic if you start to believe that, in general, relationships can't be empowering. The right relationships will not require you to surrender your power but will encourage you to embrace it more fully; they will make you feel free.

Your closest relationships should be safe spaces where you can dream and share your aspirations without fear of judgment, and where you're encouraged to pursue your visions, no matter how big or incomprehensible they may seem at first. You might feel discouraged if you share your visions with loved ones only to be routinely shut down or dismissed. It is not realistic to expect everyone will understand your visions, but it's important that you feel comfortable—and even inspired—to share them. It's already too easy for you to talk yourself out of ideas that are meant to be pursued; you don't need those close to you to talk you out of them too. Unless you request guidance, others should allow you the freedom to explore your path and come to your own answers without trying to influence you. You are here to discover your way, not to be directed by others.

Feeling respected as you make bold moves and pursue new directions will ensure that your relationships amplify rather than dampen your dynamic energy. One client shared how her decades-long marriage left her feeling disempowered, controlled, and like a shadow of herself. It was only once she left the relationship that she woke up to her power and resolved to choose only those relationships that would embolden her going forward. As a Manifestor, it may feel inspiring to be surrounded by others who are bravely building their own worlds too.

As with career, a core value for Manifestors in relationships is freedom. Consider what freedom means to you. Perhaps it's the ability to hide away in your office and create without interruption, or to manage your finances independently. Or maybe it means traveling or going on a last-minute weekend trip with friends without asking for permission, confident that your partner won't feel a hint of resentment. Maybe it involves maintaining a vibrant social life outside of your primary relationship. Freedom will look different for everyone, but having it is essential for all Manifestors. One Manifestor client expressed appreciation for her relationship dynamic, saying, "I love that I don't need to ask my husband's permission to go on trips or sign up for classes—I just inform him of my plans." Another shared, "It's beautiful to have so much freedom in a relationship and still choose each other every day."

It's no surprise that as a lover of freedom, you may have a taste for spontaneity and adventure in your relationships and appreciate those who love jumping in and experiencing new things with you. One client shared, "I love when friends come along with me on my escapades—whether it's an impromptu taco run at 2:00 a.m. or traveling across Europe for three months. And if they can't join, they encourage me to go do it on my own."

Time to be alone is also a necessity for Manifestors. It's important that those close to you don't interpret your need for solitude as a personal rejection but, rather, as a healthy expression of your independence, which gives them space to enjoy their own pursuits as well. One client shared how she loves that her partner accepts that she doesn't want to spend all their time together, but is enthusiastic when she does want a date or quality time. Honoring your need for space might look like having designated solo time on a regular basis, the freedom to let someone know when you need a guilt-free break from them, sleeping alone, or even maintaining your own home or apartment if you crave that level of personal space. Regardless of your living arrangements with a partner, having the opportunity to unwind alone at day's end can be crucial. This might feel much more natural for you than socializing or working up to the point when you go to bed.

The need for space doesn't disappear if you become a parent; if anything, it becomes even more vital. Make sure you take that time, whether it's a full evening or just ten minutes. It's also important to feel permission to approach parenting in a way that feels true to you, even if it's unconventional. You are, by design, unconventional. If you're parenting with another person, ensure they respect your approach, even if it's different from their own.

This need for independence extends to how your energy flows. Your energy naturally comes in waves, and you are at your best in relationships when you show up when the energy is there and withdraw to recharge when it is not, communicating your availability along the way. Your energy pattern—intense bursts of activity followed by periods of rest—cannot be scheduled or planned in advance. It's crucial that you feel supported to seize these bursts of energy and creativity and, also, to rest afterward without judgment. In an ideal world, others are comfortable with you opting out and being less accessible at some points than at others; they are secure and know you will return when your energy allows. If others expect constant availability, it can lead to disappointment and frustration. While some people have a steady supply of energy to expend daily, you are not built this way.

It can feel deeply nourishing when the people in your life support your natural energy cycles—whether you're in a burst of inspiration or need rest. This might be a partner bringing you snacks without the expectation of conversation during a creative surge, or handling household chores when you're in a rest cycle. It could also look like a friend sending a note saying they're excited to see what you're creating without expecting a response.

Manifestor energy is typically more closed-off, selective, and protective than that of other Types. You may struggle if you try to be open and available to everyone when you are only meant to be available for a select few, or if you take others' rejection or discomfort with your direct nature personally. The more unapologetic and authentic you are, the more you make yourself available for the right relationships, and the more you will naturally push away those who are not meant for you. One Manifestor client realized it was only when she released the need to please that she started finding people who truly resonated with her. It may feel especially validating when the people you *have* chosen to let into your life recognize how sacred it is to step into your powerful energy field. While you might not require frequent words of affirmation in the way Projectors appreciate, an occasional accolade reminding you of your impact can make you feel respected and inspire you to keep creating and showing up as yourself. One Manifestor client shared how meaningful it was when her friend sent her a note saying what a privilege it was to be her cheerleader and champion.

If a relationship brings you peace and freedom, it's a signal that the relationship is right for you. The opposite is true when a relationship regularly triggers anger, which is often a sign you lack freedom and autonomy within the relationship, and a change may be needed.

A Room of Her Own

As soon as Katy sat down, it was clear something was off.

"I'm feeling confused about my relationship," she said, tossing her short brown hair. "My boyfriend and I have been great for two years, but ever since we moved in together, I feel constricted, like I'm expected to be with him constantly. I'm not sure if this pressure is self-imposed or coming from him."

It made sense that Katy was struggling. Manifestors thrive on autonomy, and now this integral element of herself felt compromised. Since this was a new feeling, it seemed the issue might not be the relationship itself but the living situation.

"How about we think through some ways to reintroduce that sense of independence into your living arrangement?" I asked. "Maybe establishing specific times for personal space, or even discussing the idea of separate bedrooms could help."

Katy's eyes lit up at the suggestion.

"It's funny you mention that," she said. "I've always wanted my own sleeping space in a relationship but I worry about upsetting my partner or making him feel rejected."

I reminded Katy she is not designed to approach relationships like others do and encouraged her to discuss the idea of separate bedrooms openly with her boyfriend. As it turned out, he was also feeling the strain of round-the-clock intimacy. They both liked the idea of sleeping separately a few nights a week and creating more space for each of them to embrace their own rhythm.

Having her own bedroom allowed Katy to regain a sense of freedom in the relationship. She felt more connected to her partner and less guilty about taking time for herself. In the end, the relationship wasn't the problem; it was about adapting their living situation to better meet their needs. Human Design helped Katy find an approach to cohabitation that felt far more authentic and empowering to her than the "norm."

Practices

If you find yourself feeling angry or disempowered, these practices will help you regain your power and peace, both at work and within your relationships. If you already feel peaceful and free, they can dial up your impact and freedom in new, inspiring ways.

1. **Experiment with honoring the natural cycles of your energy.**

    Intense periods of action and inspiration are meant to be followed by quieter periods of rest and restoration. You are not designed to maintain consistent momentum or productivity, nor are you meant to be always available.

    Experiment with taking advantage of the energy and inspiration when it comes, and then resting once that energy starts to dwindle. Rest is not only a way to restore but, just as importantly, a space for new ideas to emerge. Because new ideas are often born in the quiet, a lack of rest can make you unavailable when new inspirations would normally arrive—or they may come, but you could miss them. If you can't practice this during the week, try integrating it into your weekends or even into a couple-hour block. Honoring your rhythms means doing what you truly have the energy for, not showing up just because you think you should.

    Sharing your energy patterns with collaborators, friends, family members, and partners can also help them better understand and respect your energy. If you work within a team, perhaps you suggest working from home every couple of weeks to have space to honor your natural energy flow. Or if you are in a romantic partnership, make it a practice to give them a heads-up whenever you feel compelled to pull back and take time away to recharge alone. Know that your collaborators and friends are likely to catch on quickly, realizing how much more impactful and happier you are when you have the freedom to operate in cycles.

2. **Share yourself in the boldest, most authentic way possible, and see who stays by your side.**

    The more you embrace your biggest, bravest self, the more you make yourself available to impact and connect with the right people: those who are naturally expanded by your presence. Dimming your light to try to fit in only makes it harder for others to support you and truly understand who you are.

    Share your grand visions in a way that feels true to you and see what happens. Who supports you? Who drifts away? Who encourages your dreams? Who shuts them down? Who inspires you to keep sharing? Who discourages you from following what feels right? This is a simple yet powerful way to connect with people who will propel you forward rather than hold you back.

3. **Consider what would make you feel the most free.**

Think about what would fulfill your need for freedom and autonomy in your relationships and at work. Is it having one set meeting a day with your team rather than being expected to be always responsive and on call? Is it reserving an afternoon each week for yourself? Is it dedicating mornings to being in your own flow? Is it having your own office or bedroom to retreat to? Is it taking a spontaneous solo trip? Or perhaps, is it informing others when you need space in real time?

Whatever it is, start making this practice—if possible—a guilt-free part of your routine, and observe how it impacts your well-being and relationships with others.

Journal Prompts

Where in your life do you feel most peaceful, empowered, and free?

Do you take rest when you're tired, or do you push yourself to keep going? Why? When are you most effective?

If you could delegate daily tasks, where would you begin?

Do you feel safe sharing your big, bold visions in your relationships? If yes, how does that feel? If not, why? Do you wish you could?

Do you feel free to take alone time without guilt in your relationships? If yes, what benefits does it bring you? If not, why, and is that something you want?

KEY INSIGHTS

PERCENT OF POPULATION	1
TRADEMARK	Objectivity
GIFTS	Feeling into a person or situation to understand what is happening in a way no one else can, showing us what's going on in our communities and spaces, being an objective observer, offering profound insights, expressing yourself in diverse ways
CHALLENGES	Being in spaces or on timelines that do not work for your sensitive and fluctuating energy, confusing the energy of others with your own, not taking sufficient time for yourself, trying to show up consistently day after day, searching for your single purpose
POPULAR ROLES	Facilitator, mediator, advisor, coach, counselor, consultant, chief of staff, artist, activist, founder, editor, investor, human resources specialist, organizational development expert, curator, interior designer
RELATIONSHIP NEEDS	Freedom to take time alone without guilt, respect for your fluctuating energy levels, appreciation of your versatile nature, recognition of your sensitivity to your surroundings, honesty

Reflector

WHEN HER HUSBAND, JIMMY, DECIDED TO RUN FOR GOVERNOR OF Georgia, Rosalynn Carter was determined to meet voters and understand what mattered most to the people of the Peach State.

One day on the campaign trail, an exhausted cotton mill worker shared that she and her husband worked opposite shifts to care for their daughter, who struggled with mental illness. It was the late 1960s, and the perception of mental health in America was markedly different from what it is today. Often labeled as "crazy," people struggling with mental health issues were forced to navigate their troubles alone or were institutionalized with very little middle ground.

Haunted by the story of the mill worker's daughter, Rosalynn urged Jimmy to prioritize mental health awareness during his campaign speeches, believing it would resonate with voters. The shift proved to be a winning strategy, as Jimmy Carter won by a landslide.

Six years after winning the governor election, when he was elected president of the United States, Jimmy Carter named Rosalynn Carter the chair of the newly formed President's Commission on Mental Health, which brought mental health activism to the forefront of American life.

In a statement released by the Carter Center upon her passing in 2023, Jimmy Carter wrote, "Rosalynn was my equal partner in everything I ever accomplished. She gave me wise guidance and encouragement when I needed it."

She was a keen observer—the kind of person who could take the temperature of any situation, reflect back what was really happening, and offer wisdom when it mattered.

That's because Rosalynn Carter was a Reflector.

At Work

As a Reflector, you are meant to wear many hats over the course of your career and to shapeshift in small and big ways. While many of us show up in more fixed, consistent ways as time goes on, Reflectors are the opposite. You tend to find success when you allow yourself to continually evolve in your work according to what feels aligned in each phase of life, instead of staying with something out of obligation or because it's what you've always done.

You might find you are sensitive to others' energy—their emotions, stress, fears, opinions, excitement about work, and beyond—often absorbing and feeling it deeply. This sensitivity allows you to understand what is happening in a team or business in a way that no one else can, or in the case of Rosalynn Carter, a society. When you do not hold on to others' feelings as your own, you become a clear mirror, easily assessing what's in front of you and reflecting back what you see to show us what's happening in our communities, spaces, and teams. You have your finger on the pulse and always seem to know exactly what's going on.

This means you thrive as an evaluator or facilitator at work. Your objectivity and innate wisdom enable you to intuit what's not working and envision how things can be improved. You are at your best when valued for your ability to suggest refinements and perceive things others miss, and when you feel like a vital part of a team, community, or someone's life. This could mean offering insights as chief of staff to a CEO, coaching a client, facilitating a small group, or as an activist, holding up a mirror to societal injustice and revealing a more equitable path. Simply put, you are here to transform the world around you through how and what you see.

One client hit her stride by building a consulting practice that supported leaders in human resources, focusing on positive employee experience as the key metric for company success. She became a trusted advisor, confidante, and emotional support to leaders, the go-to person when they sensed something was wrong but couldn't pinpoint what. She explained, "I excel in human resources because I perceive what is imperceivable by most, making the implicit explicit in company culture and employee experience." Her wise, unique perspective as a Reflector made her exceptional in this role and highly sought after.

As a Reflector, you may struggle if you lose your objectivity at work by absorbing others' stress and emotions as your own until they overwhelm you and lead to burnout. Not taking enough time for yourself—which is a crucial tool for letting go of stress, emotions, and fears that aren't yours—can make work feel unsustainable. When you practice neutral observation and recognize that not all feelings you experience are your own, you may find more people seeking out your objective perspective and come to see your insights as a rare professional gift.

This sensitivity makes it important to be selective about where and with whom you work, given how much you take in from your environment. Your energy levels mirror your team's state: a motivated and excited team will energize you, whereas a team on the verge of burnout can make you feel sluggish. An inspiring environment will bring out your most productive, inspired self, whereas an environment that feels uninspiring and unhealthy can leave you feeling depleted and disconnected, negatively impacting your well-being and performance. One client shared that her career transformed when she prioritized working with those who motivated her to grow and evolve.

Not only is your energy to make things happen influenced by your environment but it is also designed to ebb and flow throughout the month rather than on a daily basis, like Projectors. One week, you may get more done than anyone else; the next, you may need more rest. Embracing your natural rhythm is key to your success. This can mean working alone when you crave space or being around others when it feels inspiring; it all depends on how you feel and what you need at any given moment. An ideal position will be flexible and allow you to freely move your energy in and out of teams and environments based on what feels right on any given day. You may thrive working with Generators or Manifesting Generators, who can offer consistent energy and presence as your energy rises and falls. It may also feel particularly harmonious to collaborate with Projectors, who see the world uniquely and ebb and flow in their energy like you.

Because you operate differently from most people—remember, you are just 1 percent of the population—the traditional methods and rules that work for others may not work for you. Consider how you naturally like to do things and how you can build those preferences into your career. You might run your business in a way that allows you to honor the natural cycles of your energy throughout the month. You might have a team manage daily operations so you can focus on where your energy leads you each day, or you might negotiate with your boss for a flexible work schedule that will allow you to choose your work environment two days a week. If you are not yet in a position where you can be flexible, consider small ways to honor the natural fluctuations of your energy and sensitivity to space, like taking a quick break for tea when you're feeling zapped, working alongside a collaborator who enlivens you, or choosing your favorite corner of the office to work from.

When considering a new role, focus on whether your collaborators and workspace feel uplifting and inspiring, whether your perspective feels valued and sought after, whether your collaborators understand your working style, the flexibility of your work schedule, how much variety the role offers, opportunities for continued evolution and growth, the ability to make a meaningful impact on the team or community, and the emphasis on your well-being.

Feeling regularly surprised is a good sign you're on the right career path. This could mean experiencing each day as fresh and exciting, being delighted by the opportunities that show up, marveling at your many expressions, being invited to share your reflections, and seeing your insights transform spaces. When frequent, surprise signals you to keep moving in that direction in your career.

If you find yourself feeling disappointed on a regular basis, view that as an invitation to check in with yourself, make necessary changes, and align with a better direction.

The less you feel a need to put a label on who you are and what you're here to do, the more full of surprise and magic your career will be. Rather than delving into many passions at once as a Manifesting Generator does, you may find each season brings a new passion or expression of self. As I often remind my Reflector clients, the key question to ask yourself when considering your next career move is not "What is your purpose?" but "What feels most like you right now?" The harder you search for a singular purpose, the more lost you will feel, whereas embracing where you are without needing to know where it's all going will set you free.

The World through New Eyes

Ellen had been working in operations at a large tech start-up for years, fulfilling whatever function was needed at the moment, whether it was stuffing gift bags for a big event, helping the product team rethink their feature set, mediating an employee dispute, or sitting in on executive meetings and sharing her perspective. Even though her role was in operations, the CEO often sought her opinions when navigating challenges or considering a new direction.

Ellen knew her insights were valuable, particularly to the CEO, and she enjoyed her work but something felt off. When I told her about Reflectors, Ellen finally discovered what the issue was: the expectation that she be constantly accessible and active was at odds with her naturally fluctuating energy. She was being pushed to *do* when her true strength was seeing, sensing, and feeling things others did not, and offering assessments of what was not working and what was necessary to ensure progress.

In Ellen's words, "I'm just not built to take action at the same pace as my colleagues, and the more I try to keep up, the more ineffective

I feel." The requirement of her daily presence at the office also felt suffocating; the environment didn't always resonate, and the lack of variety made her feel stagnant.

Throughout our sessions, Ellen began to consider the possibility of a role better suited to her nature. A few months later, after a conversation with her CEO, Ellen shifted from full-time into a consultant position—and her previous employer became her first client. Now, rather than being overwhelmed by the office's day-to-day demands, Ellen could focus her energy on helping the CEO improve team dynamics. She reduced her presence in the office to once a week and spent that day sitting in on meetings and providing insights. What was once a peripheral involvement became her central focus.

Soon, her client roster grew. Ellen began consulting for multiple companies and became a respected source of insight—the person a CEO came to when they needed an objective perspective on what was not working. She built her business around her true gift: seeing what others could not. Ellen conducted the majority of her sessions remotely so she could work from her favorite cafés and co-working spots. By taking into consideration her unique energy needs as a Reflector, Ellen redesigned her career—and her life. The best part of her journey is that Ellen now understands her current role isn't her final destination. Her purpose cannot be contained in one title and just because she's in love with something today doesn't mean she'll love it forever. Accepting this part of her design means that she'll be ready for the next chapter of her professional evolution when the time comes.

In Relationships

As a Reflector, it is important to cultivate relationships with people who appreciate how different you are and who don't expect you to conform to the norm. The people in your life—especially the ones who you actively choose to go deep with—should be genuinely curious about how you function, as they might not understand your ways right away.

You might find different friends and groups pull out different parts of your personality. With one group, a lively and playful side might show up, while a more thoughtful and reserved side might emerge with another. This is natural for Reflectors, because you have many facets that seek expression and different relationships pull out your different expressions. Spending time in diverse communities ensures you aren't limited in your expression or overly influenced by just one person's feelings and perspective. I had a client who became convinced something was wrong with her because she started to notice how differently she showed up with her family compared to how she showed up with her friends and partner. She was concerned it was a sign of inauthenticity; I reminded her it was a sign of vastness. Whenever you're in the right place with the right people, the perfect version of you will naturally come forward. Maya Angelou's words serve as a beautiful reminder for Reflectors: "Precious jewel, you glow, you shine, reflecting all the good things in the world. Just look at yourself."

Choose to surround yourself with people excited to meet and embrace new versions of you. They do not box you into a fixed identity but appreciate bearing witness to your continued evolution. They do not meet you with the expectation of "This is who you are" but with the perspective of "I can't wait to see who you become." One client wrote, "I am undefined," in her dating bio to create space for her ongoing transformation from the outset. This variability underscores the importance of being in relationships that don't demand consistency in how you show up each day, let alone over the course of your lifetime.

Given how impacted you are by your environment and the people you're with, it's important to allow yourself to be meticulous about your surroundings in relationships. Even if it feels a bit nitpicky at times, something as seemingly small as changing tables at a restaurant is essential if the energy feels off. Your partners and friends can support you by checking in with your comfort level in new spaces, and asking questions like: Do you like the vibe of this restaurant? How does this hotel room feel? Does this neighborhood feel like one you'd want to wake up in? Those nearest and dearest to you should be happy to help you in this way because they understand that the right environment improves your experience and theirs because they receive the best of you in the right space.

Your sensitivity extends beyond space to people, which means it's essential to consider how it feels to be around someone when assessing new relationships. If a friend is enthusiastic about what they're working on, their enthusiasm will spill over to you. If a partner is stagnant in their career, you might feel that stagnation. If your sister's emotions are unexpressed, you, too, will feel heavy and tight. Invest in people who are aware of their energy impact, who take good care of their energy, and whose energy you enjoy taking in.

Be mindful that the people who feel right will evolve as you do. You might find that a group that felt like your soul family a year ago no longer feels right, or that you feel better seeing a friend you used to see daily less frequently now. Regularly take stock of where your energy feels drawn, and accept that your preferences and desires for connection will shift over time. Of course, you will have some relationships that are obligatory. In this kind of relationship, setting clear boundaries around your participation and allowing yourself time to recharge after time spent together is a healthy way to take care of yourself.

Even in the most supportive relationships, it's important to take time alone to recenter and release what's not yours. You should feel free to take that time whenever and however you need it. In a perfect world, a partner or friend will notice when you are burdened with carrying energy that's not your own or are overdue for a moment alone, and will encourage you to take some time to yourself, especially if you've just had a lot of social interaction. Your energy levels can also vary on a day-to-day basis. Ideally, those close to you regularly check in to understand your current availability rather than assuming it based on past patterns.

As a Reflector parent, it's especially important to make space to reset and recharge without guilt, even if it's just for five minutes. It may feel comforting to carve out an area in your home where you can retreat to, a space that feels like your sanctuary. Also, consider the places to take your children where the setting feels good to you too; this will help you show up as your best self.

If you live with a partner, sleeping separately and in your own energy every so often can be nourishing because it gives you space to reconnect to yourself. You may also feel best with bedtime rituals that allow you to unwind and ease into bed, which can be tricky if you share a room with a partner who works or remains energetic and engaged right up until bedtime. Reserving a moment to yourself at the day's end could benefit you both, allowing each of you to honor your own rhythm.

Whether it is a bedtime routine or another part of your life, you can feel disconnected and out of sync with your true nature if you subscribe to others' approaches in relationships over your own. Invest in relationships that respect your individuality, allow you to do things your way, and regularly surprise you with new levels and layers.

Roomie Blues

Brooke's aunt gifted her a Human Design session as a college graduation present. Brooke knew little about what to expect from our time together. It is always a gift to introduce someone to Human Design so early in their journey. Many of my clients wish they'd discovered it decades earlier.

Brooke had just moved to Los Angeles to jumpstart her career. Like many of her friends, she found a roommate on Craigslist. As soon as we sat down, Brooke began to share her concerns about her new living situation.

"I'm constantly on edge," Brooke began. "My roommate is nice, but we don't click, which makes it hard to share the same space. I need my space clean for my mental well-being, but no matter how many times we talk about it, she leaves clutter everywhere. I feel confined to my tiny room because the common spaces stress me out. I cherish my time alone because the world is a lot. But my roommate barges into my space and doesn't understand my desire for solitude. She also gets upset when I don't want to go out late with her. Sometimes I'm up for it but not always."

Her question was simple: "Should I just suck it up? Is this what living with someone in my twenties is supposed to be like?"

I love it when people intuitively express their design without knowing it.

"Brooke, it sounds like your needs are not being met in this living situation, and your design sheds some light on why," I told her. "You're right; you *are* highly sensitive to your space, and it's important that your living space feels like a sanctuary. Alone time isn't just a preference for you; it's essential. You feel the world more intensely than most, and solitude is where you recharge. Plus, your energy naturally fluctuates, which is something not everyone understands. Honoring your energetic availability moment to moment helps prevent burnout."

Brooke felt validated. The challenges she was experiencing were real. No wonder living with this roommate felt so hard. Human Design did what it so often does: it gave her the permission she needed to be herself.

After our conversation, Brooke sat down with her roommate to express her boundaries and what she needed to feel supported, but unfortunately, her roommate still didn't get it. Eventually, Brooke moved out and took her time finding a new living situation with someone who respected her needs from the start. Once she did, she was able to settle into Los Angeles and start building a life she felt comfortable in, resting easy in the fact that she finally had a nurturing environment to return to at the end of the day.

Practices

If you find yourself often feeling disappointed and disconnected, these practices can help you realign with your optimal way of operating at work and in relationships. And if your days already feel full of surprise and recognition, these practices can help ensure they stay that way.

1. **Begin each day by deciding what type of energy feels best to you.**

   What you have the energy for may vary from week to week, day to day, or even hour to hour; this is perfectly normal. Rather than waking up each day and expecting to have the same energy as yesterday, assess how you're feeling. Some days, you may feel inspired to be around others; others, you might want to be alone. Some days, you're incredibly efficient and accomplish more than anyone else; on other days, even the smallest tasks feel daunting.

   Consider how you can design a schedule that allows you to be in different environments with different people depending on how you feel that day, then adjust your to-do list and plans depending on your energy levels. If you are expected to show up the same way day after day and have little flexibility to change that, give yourself grace in the moments when your energy dwindles, knowing this is not an indicator that something is wrong with you; it's simply a reminder of your natural cycles.

2. **Practice neutral observation.**

   You are deeply sensitive and easily pick up on others' passions, fears, and feelings. This can be overwhelming if you mistake others' feelings with your own. However, this sensitivity can become a powerful asset if you learn to stay detached and not absorb the feelings around you.

   Start to practice neutral observation: sensing where others are without making it about you or taking ownership. Begin to view your feelings as intel on your environment rather than automatically assuming they belong to you or are yours to deal with. If you feel overwhelmed or unsettled in a new space, step away to reconnect to your own energy and see if the feeling lingers. Ask yourself: Is this feeling mine? Often, the question alone reveals the answer.

   Once grounded in your objectivity, share what you perceive with others if you feel inspired and invited to do so. Your ability to offer an objective perspective may lead others to seek out your insights, and sharing them can bring you purpose, energy, and inspiration.

3. Take regular time for yourself, away from others.

Your openness to those around you is a beautiful quality, but it requires that alone time be built into your life. This time will help you recenter in your energy and discern which feelings and energies are yours and which belong to others, like a friend's excitement for a new project or their stress about work.

Making solitude a regular part of your routine allows you to engage more authentically at work and in relationships, ensuring your commitments come from a genuine place. It helps you recognize your own feelings and teaches you to communicate the importance of space to those you care about. This helps them realize that your need for alone time isn't a reflection on them; it's a vital aspect of your well-being.

Journal Prompts

Where do you feel most free to do things your way rather than conform to others' approaches? How does that feel?

What direction feels most aligned to your career right now, and why?

Do you honor the natural fluctuations of your energy, or do you push yourself to keep a steady, consistent pace at work? Which approach feels better, and why?

In which relationships can you take time for yourself without guilt? How do those relationships make you feel, and why?

Who brings out a version of yourself you love, and why? Who no longer feels good to be around even if they once did?

2

Strategy

How You Create Opportunities

- Strategy is the roadmap to how you best interact with the world.

- It offers insights into how your most meaningful relationships and ideal job opportunities come about, how to be proactive in creating more of them, as well as the most effective way to communicate and connect with others.

- There are four Strategies, each linked to a Type. Generators and Manifesting Generators share the Strategy of Wait to Respond. Projectors' Strategy is to Wait for an Invitation. Manifestors' Strategy is to Initiate and Inform. Reflectors' Strategy is to Wait a Lunar Cycle.

KEY INSIGHTS

TRADEMARK	Magnetism
GIFTS	Attracting people and opportunities when you're energized and fulfilled, trusting your natural response to guide you
CHALLENGES	Fixating on a specific outcome and becoming blind to other opportunities coming your way, fearing nothing will come if you don't chase, choosing what you think you should do over what feels right, second-guessing your instinct, feeling pressured to act immediately
WORK NEEDS	Time to do what satisfies you daily, freedom to release commitments that drain you, respect for your instinctive response even when unexpected, clear yes-or-no questions for decision-making
RELATIONSHIP NEEDS	Patience with your process, recognition of your natural enthusiasm (or lack thereof), no pressure to act prematurely or explain your instincts, encouragement to follow what feels right

Wait to Respond

WHEN OPRAH WINFREY WAS OFFERED THE JOB OF HOSTING *A.M. Chicago*, a struggling morning talk show, she jumped at the chance. At the time, she was thirty years old, working on a popular show in Baltimore called *People Are Talking*, but something about it just didn't feel right. Despite many of her friends and colleagues advising her to continue building her career in Baltimore, Oprah knew she had to take the leap.

Moving to Chicago proved to be a pivotal decision in Oprah's career. The once-faltering show quickly became the highest-rated talk show in Chicago, achieved national syndication, and eventually transformed into *The Oprah Winfrey Show*, where she reinvented the talk-show format and shifted pop culture in immeasurable ways.

Just a year after making the move, Steven Spielberg caught an episode and offered her the role of Sofia in his adaptation of *The Color Purple*, which earned her an Oscar nomination and a spotlight on the international stage.

In 2011 Oprah reflected on her career in her eponymous magazine, *O*: "For all the major moves in my life—to Baltimore, to Chicago, to own my show, and to end it—I've trusted my instincts. I take in all the information I can gather. I listen to proposals, ideas, and advice. Then I go with my gut, what my heart feels most strongly."

By waiting for life to present opportunities and trusting her instincts to know which ones to pursue, Oprah Winfrey embodies the essence of her Wait to Respond Strategy as a Generator.

At Work

When you're engaged in work that excites you, your energy is naturally magnetic, pulling people and opportunities to you. Because of this, your Strategy is to wait for something to appear in your world—a text message, an idea you hear on a podcast, a tidbit that comes up in conversation, or a possible collaborator. When the right opportunity comes along, your gut will light up in response; you will feel an expansion in your belly and a literal pull. This sensation is your gut signaling you to pursue that opportunity. The more you trust this natural response, as Oprah did with the Chicago job offer, the more energy you'll have, and the more promising your opportunities will be.

Even though your powerful energy and capacity as a Generator or Manifesting Generator may tempt you to act immediately, waiting for your natural gut response helps you set boundaries and tune into what you actually have the energy for. As powerful as you are, the right action is born from receptivity and response. You might not know how something will make you feel or if you have the energy for it until it appears in your world. An external cue and an inner spark within are the surest ways to know whether a commitment is right for you.

However, this does not make responding a passive Strategy. You can actively make yourself available for better opportunities in three ways. First, do something that brings you satisfaction daily. When you are feeling regularly frustrated or dissatisfied, it's hard to attract new opportunities your way, or you may end up attracting more of what you don't want. Whereas when you are enlivened by how you're using your energy, you can't help but draw more fitting opportunities your way. As Oprah reminds us, "Life is reciprocal: the energy you expand always comes back."

Second, release commitments you no longer have the energy for. Letting go of what's no longer for you creates space for more fulfilling opportunities to show up.

Third, expand your awareness and notice what's around you. Focusing too intently on a specific outcome, like where a job might lead or landing a promotion, can prevent you from seeing the opportunities that are right in front of you simply because your attention is elsewhere.

One of my clients discovered this firsthand. Whenever her business slowed down, she felt the pressure to fill the space and come up with her next idea out of thin air. Yet she soon realized that ideas born from this pressure rarely amounted to much and only led to burnout. By waiting for ideas to emerge naturally—often inspired by a conversation or a client's suggestion—and for her gut to respond positively before pursuing them, she found herself committing to ideas that actually worked and that she had the energy to show up for. Waiting for her gut to light up before making moves was uncomfortable yet fruitful. Put another way, she found success when she trusted her natural magnetism, broadened her awareness, and stopped forcing action before the inspiration was there.

The most important piece to understand about this Strategy is that you are *always* responding: to the stores you walk by, the headlines you scroll through, and the people you see. You can respond to anything that either directly or indirectly shows up in your world. In terms of career, it might be an offer to collaborate on a project, a job posting you stumble across, or even a potential client that comes across your Instagram feed. A response can be positive, negative, or neutral. A positive response might manifest as a feeling of expansion, excitement, or a physical draw to something. A negative response could feel like a contraction, discomfort in your belly, or fatigue. A neutral feeling often appears as indifference.

For example, I have a client who plans high-end weddings. When she receives an email from a potential client, she always checks in to see if she feels excited about the prospect of the project. If she decides to move forward to a discovery call, she checks her gut again: Does she feel more energized than she did when the call started? Or does she feel depleted? She knows whether or not a potential client is the right fit based on these cues. Like this client, it's not about figuring out what you think you want but paying attention to what your body naturally responds to.

I once had a session with someone who had a vision for her dream client. Since she knew exactly who her prototype was, she figured she could easily go out and find them. Yet her business hit roadblock after roadblock no matter how hard she pushed and how many potential clients she pitched. In the midst of her frustration, she attended a weekend conference. As she shared her business struggles, a fellow attendee suggested she consider specializing in LinkedIn marketing—a concept she had never thought of but felt instantly drawn to. Inspired by this nudge from her gut, my client returned to the drawing board and rebuilt her entire business, focusing on this newfound direction. And no surprise, it worked. That was three years ago. Last week, one of my students happened to ask me, "Have you heard about this teacher? I just signed up for her course to learn how to market on LinkedIn." You guessed it: the teacher my student was talking about was my former client.

Another client told me about the time she got fired up after reading an article in the *Wall Street Journal*. She felt like something was missing and was driven to fix it. Following this natural response, she reached out directly to the editor to share her thoughts about what could be improved. That outreach led to a monthslong collaboration on multiple pieces.

In both of these instances, something unexpected showed up, their gut responded, and they followed it. This is what it looks like to respond. Notice how both of these moments could be easily dismissed if they hadn't been attuned to or trusted their natural responses. Your gut response acts as a kind of radar, indicating when it's time to pursue something. While waiting for a response is an integral part of your Strategy, your gift actually lies in action; waiting simply ensures that action is directed toward making the *right things* happen.

With this Strategy, you may also find that you respond best to specificity rather than open-ended questions. For example, you may find yourself lost in a world of endless possibilities if someone asks, "What do you want to do next in your career?" Conversely, if someone asks, "Do you want to pursue this opportunity or that one?" it's likely far easier to drop out of your head and into your gut, where the answer lies. I once had a client faced with two exciting opportunities but unsure of which to go after. So, I asked: "Does the timing feel right to pursue this one?" He responded with a resounding yes. When I posed the same question about the other opportunity, he gave a definitive no. The specificity of the questions immediately brought the clarity he was seeking. It can be that simple.

Specific questions are a tool that will serve you well when you're on the job too. This might look like requesting that collaborators offer you two potential options to choose from rather than working through a series of open-ended questions when you need to solve the problem on the spot. This can make professional conversations and decisions feel efficient and effective rather than draining and never-ending.

Manifesting Generators specifically may find it helpful to not only pay attention to the visceral response to what shows up but also to then visualize the possibility of actually making that thing happen. If your gut lights up in response to the opportunity *and* the visualization, you have the double confirmation you need that it's the right thing to pursue. If your gut reacts positively to the opportunity but not to the visualization of it, it's not the right time to commit.

As a Generator or Manifesting Generator, the belief that you must chase and create opportunities through sheer determination might be deeply ingrained. You may fear that waiting for things to unfold naturally will lead to missed chances or nothing happening at all. Yet still, I invite you to try on the idea, just for a moment, that waiting for your body to light up in response to opportunities, rather than pursuing what you think you should do, is the most reliable path to ensure you use your precious energy wisely and well. This is not to say your mind isn't powerful, because it is. But your mind is meant to be a source of inspiration and insight for others rather than a tool for solving the puzzle of your own life. That role belongs to your gut.

Poet Rumi said it best: "When I run after what I think I want, my days are a furnace of stress and anxiety; if I sit in my own place of patience, what I need flows to me."

From Dark to Light

Andi had just started a new job that, by all measures, felt like her dream job. She had envisioned this specific position for five years before landing the exact role she had been dreaming of. The only problem was that, once she actually started working in the position, she disliked everything about it. The work was dull, her collaborators were uninspired, and she felt unmotivated—a far cry from the passion and drive she normally brought to her work.

She took our call from a room so dark that I could barely see her face. The darkness seemed to mirror the state she was currently in: frustrated, confused, and lost.

"I chased what I thought was my dream career," she said, shaking her head, "only to despise it once I landed it. Why? This job ticked every box on my list. The salary is competitive, the commute is short, and honestly, as silly as it sounds, it seems impressive to my friends and family."

Without looking at her chart, it was evident that Andi's pursuit of the "perfect job" was shaped more by what she *thought* she should want than by true excitement.

Looking at Andi's Strategy, we discovered that the right opportunities for her were not meant to be forced. Instead, they were the ones that showed up in her world and just *felt* right, even if they weren't what she might have predicted. The misalignment with her Strategy became clear as we talked.

"Andi, how did it feel when you were offered the position?" I asked.

"It didn't feel right. Looking back, I felt so swayed by my idealized vision for my career that I prioritized that over what felt right in my gut."

Despite her frustration at finding herself in the wrong job, Andi felt relieved to understand why her "dream job" didn't feel like such a dream after all.

Soon after our session, Andi left her job. Thankfully, she had saved enough money to be able to leave her current position even without another lined up.

"Try this," I suggested when we spoke next. "Release the vision of what your perfect role is supposed to look like. Instead, make it your job to use up your energy in ways that you enjoy on a daily basis. Trust that this will pull the most aligned opportunities your way. Then, pay attention to what comes into your life and feels right in your gut. Your mind won't stop getting in the way, so the work here is to trust how your gut responds to what shows up rather than listening to the *should*s in your mind."

Andi went all in on the new approach. She filled her days talking to past colleagues and friends who inspired her, moved her body in ways that energized her, and made space for passions she had previously deemed unimportant.

Within three weeks, a friend mentioned a new opportunity at a healthcare start-up to Andi as the two were enjoying a casual cup of coffee. The job diverged from Andi's initial aspirations but instinctively felt right.

This time, Andi chose to trust her intuition.

I continued to work with Andi for several more years and, as time passed, our sessions moved from dark rooms to sunlit ones. Over time, I watched her build an extraordinary team at that healthcare start-up, have a powerful impact introducing a groundbreaking product to the market, and ultimately transition out of that role to work for herself. Appropriately, Andi's new gig involves supporting executives in finding more fulfillment in their careers and lives.

In the end, Andi's career unfolded in a deeply satisfying way because she stopped trying to force her next step and what she thought she should want into existence. Instead, she paid attention to what showed up and felt right, trusting that one aligned step after another would take her in the perfect direction.

How Do You Choose?

In Relationships

Just as you are meant to follow your natural response when choosing a career path, you are meant to do the same in your relationships. When starting new relationships, pay attention to who you naturally feel drawn to, not who you think you should like or be friends with. You might have an idea of your ideal partner or friend, only to be surprised that someone else resonates more.

Whose energy makes you feel expansive and excited? Who makes you contract and pull away? Your body instinctively knows who's right for you, and deepening your attention to its innate response can help you more quickly and easily find your way into the best relationships. This might look like seeing someone's profile on a dating app and feeling your whole body light up in response or noticing someone across the room and feeling a strong pull toward them for no apparent reason. You may notice that conversations flow comfortably and freely when you feel instinctively drawn to someone. On the other hand, if you're not pulled toward a person but think you should be, the conversation may feel forced and stunted. If you ignore the nudges you feel to explore certain people or conversations, you might miss out on unexpectedly meaningful relationships. You may convince yourself it doesn't make sense to reach out to that person or talk to that stranger, when they might just become your dream collaborator, friend, or even partner. Your nudges guide you to the right people; your job is simply to trust them.

Sometimes, your natural response may be immediate. One client instantly knew her future husband was the one even though he looked nothing like she expected. Sure enough, just three months after meeting, they were married.

"It took me thirty-seven years," she said, "but I finally found him."

Another client randomly met his wife halfway around the world when he wasn't even looking to date. His brain said no, but his body said yes. Eight years and many flights later, they are still happily together.

Other times, you may feel drawn to someone, but the timing doesn't feel right. One client first met her partner through events she organized when she was nineteen. Both were in relationships when they met, yet she remembers being pulled to him from the moment she saw him. He felt the same. Years passed without contact, but they followed each other's lives from afar. A year ago, they matched on a dating app while he was visiting her hometown; she swiped right, and so did he. The moment they reconnected, they felt the same draw toward one another, and the timing finally felt right. They've been together ever since.

The pull you feel toward someone should continue over time, so it's important to stay connected to how your body responds throughout the duration of a relationship. One client who has been married for nineteen years says that she continues to feel a full-bodied yes and a deep excitement every time her husband asks her out.

If you feel there's an absence of good relationships in your life, focus on using your energy in ways that bring you joy. When you feel fulfilled by your daily activities, such as working at a job you love or moving your body in ways that revitalize you, the people who enter your life will often resonate more deeply than those who show up when you're feeling frustrated and drained. How fantastic is that? You get to make yourself available for better relationships by enjoying yourself more. One client shared that in her forty-one years of dating, it was during the two time periods when she felt most content and satisfied with life that she met both her ex-husband and husband. Once she reached those high points, it only took a matter of weeks for her partners to appear. You may struggle if you initiate relationships for fear that no one will show up in your life rather than trusting that the right ones will arrive when you're doing what you love.

Bear in mind that your Strategy of responding also applies to choosing the mechanisms through which you meet people. If dating apps exhaust you, they may not be right for you. If meeting people in person feels expansive and exciting, focus on that instead.

Just like in your career, when making decisions, you thrive in your personal life when given specific options as opposed to open-ended questions. It's important that the people you're in relationships with know this so they can present options, like suggesting dinner possibilities instead of asking you what you want to eat. If you don't communicate your need for clear options to respond to, you may feel indecisive when people ask you an open-ended question you don't have an immediate answer to. It's not that you're indecisive; you just need specific communication that drops you into your gut and draws the answers out of you. You might feel particularly supported when the people in your life pay attention to your visceral response to what is presented and recognize the difference between when you are speaking from a place of genuine excitement versus one of obligation, overwhelm, or exhaustion. When your loved ones are attuned to you in this way, they can remind you of your natural response in the moments when you forget. It is also important your visceral responses are taken seriously even when they don't align with what others want from you.

All of this means it's important to stay connected to your instinctive response in relationships rather than overthinking, people-pleasing, or obsessing about what you should do. For instance, don't force difficult conversations just because you think you should; wait until it feels right. Or if someone suggests moving in together, notice how your body feels about it rather than immediately trying to rationalize the decision or running through a list of pros and cons. Putting too much focus on others' needs or overthinking what you *should* want can cause unnecessary challenges and lead you to make the wrong commitments. The more you allow yourself to be in the moment and tune into what your body has to say, the more you and your relationships will thrive.

Letting Go of the List

Josh felt alone and frustrated when it came to dating. Everyone around him seemed happily partnered, yet he remained unsure of how to find a fulfilling relationship. He wanted to know why dating felt so hard for him and, by that point, was open to any modality that might provide insight. Human Design was his last resort.

First, I needed to know how Josh had been approaching dating up to this point. He explained, "I have a very specific vision of the partner

I'm seeking, and my standards are high. Nobody is showing up who checks all the boxes, so I'm not pursuing anyone. I don't feel like anyone who shows up is even close to a good fit."

Human Design often suggests an approach quite different from what we've tried before, and Josh was no exception. I warned Josh that he might not resonate with what I shared, and that was perfectly okay.

"You're not meant to construct a vision of your ideal partner and then find them. Instead, you're meant to pay attention to who shows up in your world and who you naturally respond to. The person may not always be who you expect. Follow who your body responds to, not who your mind thinks you should pursue." I took a beat and then continued. "Also, it's hard to attract the right people when you feel unfulfilled and annoyed by your day-to-day life. How do you feel about your life in general? Are you excited by how you're using your energy, or do you spend a lot of time exhausted and irritated?"

Josh nodded knowingly. He acknowledged that his dating dry spell had just so happened to coincide with a very frustrating period at work. He was in a job he disliked and spent most of his time bemoaning how awful it was. While Josh wasn't ready to completely commit to letting go of his list, he did agree to give it a try given that his current approach wasn't working.

After our session, Josh's first step was simply to use his energy in a more satisfying way. For him, that meant picking one of his favorite activities, rock climbing, back up, which he had stopped due to work stress. He also made a point of reconnecting with friends he loved but hadn't seen much recently.

At first, Josh's dating life didn't change much, but he did begin to feel better, lighter, and more satisfied on a day-to-day basis. Then, a few months later, he sent me a note letting me know he'd met a man at his rock-climbing gym who didn't fit one of the most fundamental criteria on his list: instead of pursuing a traditional nine-to-five career like Josh had always assumed his future partner would—and like Josh himself had—he was an artist. Still, the man felt right in ways Josh couldn't explain. He decided to let his body lead this time.

With his trusty list in hand, Josh never would have pursued this man, but when he let his gut lead, he couldn't deny how right it felt. Soon, they began dating seriously.

Practices

If you find yourself chasing opportunities and relationships more often than attracting them, adopting the following practices can be an impactful way to experiment with your Strategy. If ample opportunities and people are already flowing your way, these practices will only heighten their quality.

1. **Pursue what you feel naturally excited by without knowing where it will take you.**

    You might often feel drawn to people, opportunities, and places without knowing why. For instance, you might want to pursue a master's in counseling without intending to become a therapist, go to culinary school in Paris just because, or feel an inexplicable pull to move to the woods and grow your own food despite the fact that it seems illogical.

    Trust that your natural response will guide you to where you need to be. Whatever captures your interest has a purpose, even if the purpose is not clear yet. Your job is to follow these hints, taking the next step that feels right in your career (and life), without obsessing about the final destination. Often, the path you're naturally guided to is so much more magical and fulfilling than the one you originally planned.

2. **If you feel nothing is coming, pay attention to what is already in your orbit.**

    Take stock of what's already present in your world. You might be overlooking a possibility that has been subtly calling to you, whether it's a potential collaboration, an opportunity, a course, a friend, a romantic prospect, or a business idea.

You can also give yourself new things to respond to by putting yourself in the way of new inputs—attend events, listen to podcasts, explore job listings, or have conversations with colleagues and friends to see if anything sparks your gut. Do you feel expanded, energized, and inspired when an opportunity or person shows up? Or do you feel contracted, deflated, and exhausted?

3. **Have someone ask you specific questions about an opportunity you want clarity on.**

Specific yes-or-no questions cut through the mental clutter and direct you straight to your gut response. If you're having a hard time accessing clarity, have someone close to you pose specific questions.

These questions might include things like: *Does this job feel right? Is now the right time to pursue it? Are you excited to work with these potential colleagues? Is this the right direction for your career? Does this relationship feel right? Do you feel excited to spend more time with this person?* Pay attention to the visceral response that comes before your mind has a chance to get in the way.

Journal Prompts

What and who are you most drawn to right now?

Do you usually chase opportunities, or do they come to you? Which approach works better for you, and why?

When making decisions at work, do you prefer open-ended questions or specific options? Why?

Who notices and respects your genuine excitement about what is presented even when it doesn't align with their expectations? How does that feel, and do you want more of it?

When was a time someone didn't feel right, but you pursued the relationship anyway? What was the outcome, and what did you learn?

Wait for an Invitation

IN 1984 RUPAUL ANDRE CHARLES WAS HUSTLING HARD. AS A YOUNG artist with dreams of making it big in New York City, he was recording demos, sending out press kits, and playing live shows. But it wasn't until talent managers Randy Barbato and Fenton Bailey randomly saw RuPaul on the street pasting promotional posters of himself onto buildings that his life would change forever.

"We fell in love [with him] instantly," they reflected in an interview with *Los Angeles Magazine*. As the story goes, they introduced themselves and invited RuPaul to sign with their production company, World of Wonder Productions. RuPaul had a feeling that these guys might be his ticket to stardom, and he was right.

Once he released his debut single, "Supermodel (You Better Work)," the world found out what Barbato and Bailey knew in an instant: RuPaul was a star. The breakout hit quickly topped the charts, and over the following forty years, the two strangers who had spotted his potential on the side of the road would go on to guide his legendary career.

In addition to becoming a musical icon, RuPaul became the first openly gay host of a nationally syndicated talk show with *The RuPaul Show* and

KEY INSIGHTS

TRADEMARK	Being recognized and invited
GIFTS	Possessing unique talents that are here to be seen, invitations leading to the next step in your career and life
CHALLENGES	Trying to convince people of your value, chasing opportunities, accepting every invitation, undervaluing yourself, shying away from your gifts out of fear, offering advice without considering if it's welcome
WORK NEEDS	Opportunities to share your unique talents, feeling appreciated in a way that fuels you, confidence that your insights are desired and acted upon
RELATIONSHIP NEEDS	Thoughtful questions, words of affirmation, invitations to shared experiences, requests for your insight and advice, feeling continuously recognized for who you are and all that you can be

he won fourteen Emmy Awards for creating and starring in the smash hit reality show *RuPaul's Drag Race*, making him the most-awarded person of color in Emmy history.

All of this success came from accepting the right invitation at the right time—a perfect example of RuPaul following his Strategy of Wait for an Invitation as a Projector.

At Work

Remember that, as a Projector, you operate differently from 80 percent of the world. Your true value lies not in how much you do, but in the depth of your insights, talents, and ability to guide others toward using their energy more effectively and sustainably.

Rather than chasing after opportunities, you are designed to wait for a person or opportunity to recognize your unique value and invite you to share it. An invitation is a tool to help you assess whether an opportunity places you in a position where your gifts will truly be appreciated or risks landing you in a role that doesn't fit, like being a perpetual doer and executor.

I want to be honest: When I first discovered this was my Strategy, I couldn't envision how opportunities I was excited about could possibly find me this way. But I soon recognized the power of the invitation—it's not a restriction but a safeguard for my energy, ensuring I share my guidance, gifts, and insights only with those ready to receive them. Whether it's holding back advice until asked or saying yes only to opportunities where your talents are valued and given a platform, the invitation promises you share your gifts with those who will appreciate them. It's a tool to propel you forward, not to hold you back.

As Projectors, our energy can be intense because we see people and situations so clearly. It's tempting to share all that we see with those around us, and often, what we share will be of great benefit to others. However, if people aren't ready to hear or act on our guidance, our unsolicited advice can be unwelcome. This can leave us feeling ignored and resentful if our advice goes unheeded or is poorly received. An invitation reveals whether there's room for our contributions to be valued and taken seriously, whereas ignoring our audience's receptivity (or lack thereof) is a fast track to embitterment. For instance, if you notice something at work that could be improved, wait for an invitation to share your insights or mention to a collaborator you have some thoughts to share and ask if they're open to hearing them, instead of offering your opinion unprompted. Even then, gauge their true openness before sharing. Offering your insights only when your audience is ready makes all the difference.

An invitation can manifest in various ways: a direct offer to join a project or company, a request for your insight on a topic, or an opportunity to showcase your talents on a new stage—like when Barbato and Bailey invited RuPaul to sign with their production company. Recruiters can work well for Projectors because their entire job revolves around seeing gifts and pairing them with an environment that wants or needs them. One client shared that any time she followed a career opportunity brought to her through a recruiter, she ended up with a job offer. Invitations can come in both formal and subtle ways. The way we're defining it here, an invitation is a feeling that your talents are valued and being specifically requested, whether through a formal invitation, a subtle glance, or a question. Also keep in mind that invitations can have a shelf life. If an opportunity that once energized you now leaves you feeling drained and disillusioned, it might be time to consider moving on or having a conversation to see if the invitation still stands and you remain appreciated for what you bring.

Understand that this Strategy does not prevent you from applying for jobs or even reaching out to potential collaborators. I encourage you to apply to jobs that excite you, but I do recommend that you refrain from committing to a new opportunity unless you feel sincerely recognized and welcomed by your future colleagues. If you feel inspired to reach out to someone, consider simply making your presence and expertise known rather than overtly selling yourself. This gives others the space to respond (or not) without pressure, and provides you with a gauge of how your gifts and expertise will be received. In other words, do you feel invited once you make your presence known? The right opportunity will make you feel seen and sure that you're the person meant to fill that role.

Not all invitations will be right for you, and not all recognition is equal. For example, while you might be praised for your proficiency at a role, that doesn't necessarily mean it resonates with you or aligns with your self-perception or passions. When you feel genuinely recognized, even by just one person, it energizes you and sparks inspiration to share your talents in your professional life. True recognition makes you feel deeply and specifically seen for your distinct gifts. Without it, you will often feel a drain on your energy, and it'll be hard to muster enough energy to show up well and sustainably. This lack of recognition can leave you feeling bitter and serve to diminish your self-worth rather than affirm the importance and necessity of your talents. One coach shared how energized she felt when working with clients who treasured her perspective and how depleted she felt when coaching those who made her feel unseen and seldom acted on her insights despite hiring her to guide them. The invitation was there but the recognition was not.

If you doubt invitations will come your way, you might find yourself trying to initiate and force opportunities. It's not that opportunities can't emerge this way, but they will likely feel much harder and full of resistance when they do. You may discover the opportunities are not only bigger but also feel better when you're genuinely invited and seen from the start.

One client shared that she moved to New York City eager to enter the production industry. For two years, she chased opportunities, and it was two years of rejection and bitterness; she wondered why things weren't working out. She then started to share organically about her work on social media, and this led to an invitation from her best friend's brother to work in event production with him, which not only felt right but gave her the space and funds to set up the framework for her own business. Another friend then invited her to manage social media for their start-up.

How Do You Choose?

Though neither opportunity was what she initially envisioned, both made her feel seen and provided the resources, flexibility, and lifestyle she had been seeking.

As with all aspects of Human Design, it's best to experiment to discover what feels best for you. For instance, one client disliked the language of "waiting" and reinterpreted the invitation as choosing who and what sees him for who he authentically is. In his words, "Does this person, organization, or situation have the energetic space to receive me, and do they appreciate my specific gifts?"

It's important to note invitations are not required for everything. In the context of work, invitations matter most when sharing your gifts directly with an individual or company, and when choosing collaborators. You don't need an invitation to make art, start a business (though recognition from those you work with is key), or share your work on social media. For example, you can launch a business on your own, but if you're seeking investors, it's crucial they recognize and understand your vision. In my work, I don't need an invitation to share what I do on social media—this is a powerful strategy to gain visibility for the right recognition. However, when assessing potential partnerships, team members, or even publishing houses for this book, my guiding question is: Does this person truly understand and value what I'm doing? That's my compass. And the vast majority of the time, the people I work with are those who reached out to me.

Additionally, invitations aren't needed for every interaction or next step. What's most important is feeling invited at the start of an opportunity. Once recognized, you can freely initiate and create within that experience as long as the recognition remains.

This Strategy is not passive—none in Human Design are. While waiting for the next right invitation, focus on honing your gifts. Pay attention to what you're good at and uniquely see. When you recognize your own value at work and understand what a treasure your gifts are (beyond how much you can do), it makes it easier for others to see your gifts too.

Visibility is also key; you cannot be invited if others are unaware of your presence and talents. Instead of pitching individuals, explore broader methods to showcase your work and make your abilities known, whether through newsletters, social media, events, podcasts, or conversations with friends and colleagues. One of my Projector clients explained that he stopped focusing on perfecting his resume and, instead, started telling his network that he was looking for opportunities and getting specific about what he was looking for. In other words, he made himself visible. That's how he landed his current role.

I resisted visibility for the first two years of my business, and not co-incidentally, I struggled. Clients were hard to come by, and my business partner and I weren't earning enough to sustain the business. It was only when I overcame my fear and decided to start letting people know what I was learning and excited about—on social media, on podcasts, at events, and in casual conversations—that opportunities started to emerge. While pitching specific people never worked, sharing my work broadly without expectation always did. Researcher and storyteller Brené Brown captures it perfectly: "Courage starts with showing up and letting ourselves be seen." Trusting in the value of my work in Human Design and holding on to self-belief kept me going during the years when external recognition was scarce.

Unlike Generators and Manifesting Generators, who are waiting for something in their world to light them up whether or not it's directed at them, Projectors are waiting for someone to recognize their unique value and invite them to share it. Ultimately, as a Projector, you're not here for just any opportunity but for the right invitation that unlocks your gifts and gives them space to come alive. And you can play an active role in making that happen by making yourself visible and letting the world know that you—and your talents—exist.

For me, invitations have always taken me in a direction I would have never expected but turned out better than anything I could have imagined—like being invited to study Human Design, which revolutionized my career and life. Time and time again, invitations have served as a reliable guide to help me know who is ready for me and when, even before I know what to look out for.

The Best Medicine

Denise dialed in for our meeting from the break room of the hospital where she had dedicated the last decade to being a surgeon. She was visibly worn out from a grueling twelve-hour shift. While she felt deeply connected to her work, it was increasingly taking a personal toll. She crawled into bed bone-tired most nights, and everything else in her life had fallen by the wayside: friendships, romantic partnerships, and self-care.

As we explored her design, I asked Denise if there were aspects of her life where she felt appreciated in a way that made her feel deeply seen. She smiled.

Beyond her surgical duties, Denise served as a pillar of support for her colleagues. Despite her own challenges at work, she was passionate about helping other medical professionals navigate the system in a healthy and sustainable way, and she was the go-to person in her practice for advice and encouragement.

The day before our session, a fellow surgeon had asked Denise if she'd ever considered a role focused on supporting surgeons, expressing how valuable that type of support would be. Denise was already doing that naturally, but she'd never imagined it could be a professional path.

"Could that really be a career?" she wondered.

As we explored Denise's design, it became clear that this acknowledgment from her colleague had struck a chord. While Denise was a talented surgeon with many accolades, her career never felt like a true reflection of what she wanted to offer the world.

So, Denise decided to do something about it.

She launched a coaching practice to provide the kind of support to surgeons and healthcare providers that she found lacking in her own experience. It felt like a contribution to the medical world but in a way that was better aligned with her gifts. The colleague who made the suggestion became Denise's first client.

As a Projector, Denise has a knack for guiding others and optimizing how things are done. Her Strategy of Wait for an Invitation helped her discover the perfect way to apply these gifts to the medical system itself.

In Relationships

You bring a quality of connection not everyone is ready for, so you're meant to enter new relationships not by chasing them but by focusing on those who genuinely recognize and invite you and who are ready for the depth of connection you offer. This applies to both romantic and platonic relationships. A tough but important truth is that not everyone, even those you want to, will see you—and that's okay. The people you invest your energy in should make you feel seen and wanted; that's why the invitation is your most powerful tool for determining who is best.

When seeking new romantic partnerships or communities, start by making yourself visible—whether through dating apps, online communities, attending in-person events, or simply letting friends know you're looking. Show up courageously as yourself and pay attention to who comes to you in these environments, where the connection feels easy, natural, and authentic. You may be surprised by how magnetic your energy is to the right people. Just as in your career, visibility opens the door to aligned invitations.

An invitation into a new relationship can take many forms. It might come through someone initiating one-on-one time, asking meaningful questions, or making you feel known in a way that defies explanation. Whether it's a formal invitation or an intuitive sense of being welcomed, you'll know it when you feel it.

As a Projector, you can make the first move in a relationship if you sense genuine curiosity from someone and feel the other person leaning into the connection. The energy you bring to this kind of interaction should be about letting people know how you feel rather than pushing anything on them or expecting them to respond in a certain way. Make your feelings known and let the other person choose how to engage.

A client of mine met her fellow Projector husband at work. This now-husband wanted to date my client for years but never made a move. One day, my client's boss suggested she invite him to join a work gathering at a bar. She did and knew he was the one from the moment he walked in. Another Projector client and her Projector husband were set up by mutual friends, and both accepted the setup. While Projectors can absolutely invite others if they feel seen, these are examples of the ways in which others can step in and help initiate relationships for Projectors.

This need for invitations only pertains to the beginning of a relationship. You don't need to wait for every single social invitation once you're in a relationship. That initial recognition helps you know where to invest your energy; once you feel seen, you should feel free to pursue deepening the connection. That said, in your larger community, it may feel best when people directly invite you to participate in social gatherings and experiences, as it shows your presence is specifically desired. My favorite Projector party trick is to find a cozy, quiet spot where those interested in connecting can easily find me.

In your closest relationships, it is essential that your interactions are based on a continuous feeling of recognition and that those close to you understand your need for specific acknowledgment. Words of affirmation that highlight what someone specifically sees in you can go a long way. One mother shared how much more her recognition landed when she praised her daughter for specific actions and qualities rather than offering more general compliments. Like, "I love how you stuck up for your sister when she was feeling down," or "I loved your perspective on this; it really changed how I saw things." Another client shared that once he made an effort to recognize his partner for her distinct gifts and brave choices, she became unstoppable in her work and newly energized at home. Even though words of affirmation weren't initially natural for him, their impact undeniably fueled her with the energy to show up in their relationship and her life.

Once you're in a relationship, the invitation is also a powerful tool for communication. It's easy for you to look at someone and see their potential and all the ways they can improve their life. It's also natural that you want to share your insights immediately—trust me, I know. But if your loved ones aren't ready to hear what you have to share, your advice will fly right over their head, and you'll be left feeling unseen and resentful. Use the invitation to assess the right timing to share what you see. When people are ready, they'll ask for your input. This approach ensures your guidance is well received and that you don't come across as overly critical or as a know-it-all.

A client used to offer her younger sister advice but felt bitter when it was ignored (which was often). Meanwhile, her sister felt judged. The truth is that her sister wasn't interested in advice yet. When my client decided to wait for her sister to ask for guidance, she was able to conserve her energy and feel less resentful toward her sister. Eventually, the sister started asking for my client's input. Once she did, my client watched her advice take hold in a way it never had before she was invited to share. Another client shared that her relationships transformed when she started asking friends whether they wanted her opinion or just needed to vent. In her words, "This single-handedly changed my satisfaction with my friends. It's disempowering to think I need to wait on the sidelines to be tagged into the game. Asking the question is like ringing the doorbell to see if they want my advice."

In relationships, you may feel recognized not only when invited to share your perspective, but also when you are invited to share about your day, as well as any deeper ideas you've been pondering. It's easy for you to be pigeonholed into the role of perpetual question asker (because you are so good at it). I personally find that being on the receiving end of thoughtful questions is one of the quickest ways to feel seen in a relationship. Yes, you naturally make others feel understood, but the most fulfilling relationships are those where you also feel deeply understood, even if you initially feel vulnerable. As a Projector, don't shy away from people who see you. If you deflect others' questions and avoid sharing your true self, you deny yourself the deep connection and fulfillment that comes from being truly known—the very experience you so naturally provide to those around you. Embrace the vulnerability of being seen and allow yourself to receive the understanding you so effortlessly offer others.

How Do You Choose?

When Projector clients discuss their dissatisfaction in relationships with me, my first question is: Do you feel acknowledged and seen in this relationship? Almost always, the answer is no. If recognition or appreciation fades, it's a signal to reassess whether the relationship still feels right.

Imagine friendships and romantic partnerships in which you feel deeply wanted and known, are invited to take up space in someone's world, and have ample space to share your perspective and all that you are. This should be your standard.

From Friends to Forever

I was drawn to Jared the minute I met him. He wore a stylish gray jacket and a matching fedora, and was charismatic, hilarious, and full of life. Still, I didn't think he was my type.

Yet he kept inviting me to play a larger role in his life. First, he invited me to consult for his company. Then, we became friends, and he regularly went out of his way to spend quality time with me. As someone who tended to ask all the questions in relationships, I felt like I'd met my match in Jared. He asked question after question about my life and how I experienced the world, and he quickly got to know me on a level few have.

Before I knew it, we were best friends. Both of us are keen observers, and we loved spending time together, just taking in the world. This is not to say we are alike. We are anything but. Yet he felt like the yang to my yin.

Our friends started noticing and calling us "romantic, nonsexual best friends" because we'd never tiptoed into romance. We both had our own storied romantic histories, and we didn't want to disrupt the sanctity of our friendship.

Eventually, I realized I'd never felt more seen than I did with Jared. If he was already my favorite person, why not consider him as a romantic partner? The recognition was there, but the formal invitation was not.

I decided to share my feelings. My Strategy reminded me that pushiness never works, so trusting the genuine recognition I felt from him, I simply let him know where I stood and gave his Generator gut something to respond to.

I remember that night clearly. We were at our favorite haunt, the lights dim, sitting at our usual table.

"Jared," I said. "I'm not trying to convince you of anything. But I feel a romantic door has opened with us, and I am inspired to walk through it. If it doesn't feel right, I understand. I love being your friend. But if you're not interested only because you're scared, I will need a little space."

That directness was unusual for me, but I didn't want to be around someone making decisions out of fear when I was trying to be brave. So, without saying another word, I stood up and left the table. I had made my feelings clear, and it was up to him to respond.

The next day, he came to my apartment, and our romantic relationship began. Seven years, two dogs, one horse, and two daughters later, it is clear we made the right decision. I'm proud I trusted the energetic invitation and had the courage to share my feelings.

I offer this story as a reminder that our Strategy is meant to empower us, not limit us. For me, trusting the energetic invitation was the right choice rather than waiting for a formal one.

Practices

If you find yourself feeling bitter and chasing after opportunities and relationships that never seem to work out, these practices are a helpful way to begin to trust the power of the invitation. If you already feel appreciated at work and home, they can help you continue to practice discernment going forward.

How Do You Choose?

1. **Take the time to recognize at least one gift you bring to the table.**

   Your gift may lie in the way you make your colleagues and friends feel, the depth of your questions, your efficiency, the fresh perspective you bring, your expertise in certain processes, or your ability to communicate clearly. It doesn't matter if it's small or big; what matters is that it's a gift you bring to the world that makes you feel seen.

   As Projectors, sometimes we are so gifted at seeing others' talents but blind to our own. If you're having a hard time connecting to a gift, ask those close to you for help identifying what makes you great. Clearly seeing your own gifts and standing in your worth not only affirms your value but also helps others recognize and appreciate your contributions more clearly.

2. **Practice guiding others by asking the right questions.**

   You naturally see and feel so much, and it can be enticing to want to share everything you observe. The problem is that if people aren't ready to hear what you see, they might ignore your advice, leaving you feeling bitter and drained.

   I've found that a powerful approach to sharing information is to ask questions and then wait until the person you're speaking with directly requests advice. When you ask questions (as opposed to telling people what to do), you may find they're more receptive to your guidance. Or you can let someone know you have something you'd like to share and ask if they're open to hearing it, then check in with yourself to make sure they truly are. This ensures there is space in their energy for your wisdom to land.

3. **Consider one place to courageously make yourself visible.**

   Sharing yourself and your work with the world is scary, but it is what allows you to be seen. Consider one new place where you can make yourself visible so that you can attract the right invitations. Maybe it's launching that podcast you've dreamt about, hosting a small workshop and inviting your community, sharing your passions on Instagram, creating YouTube content, setting up a profile on a dating app, attending a social event you would not usually attend, or simply sharing your excitement about what you're working on when a friend asks.

Not everyone will connect with who you are and what you offer, and that's okay. The right people will when you show up authentically and courageously.

Journal Prompts

Where do you feel most seen? How do those places feel? How does that compare to the places where you feel overlooked?

What do you consider your greatest strengths at work, and why?

Do you actively work to make your talents visible? What happens when you do? If not, what's holding you back?

Which friends and partners ask thoughtful questions and seek your perspective? Is that something you desire more of, and why?

What actions make you feel most appreciated in your relationships, and why?

Initiate and Inform

IN 1971 GLORIA STEINEM HAD HAD ENOUGH. AFTER SERVING AS A columnist for *New York* magazine and finding that most journalism catered to men and captured women exclusively in limited and traditional roles, she had a vision: to create a publication that, as she put it, "didn't . . . just focus on women's outsides, but also our insides."

Together with activist Dorothy Pitman Hughes, she cofounded *Ms.* magazine and sparked a revolution. At a time when the media covered women as homemakers, parents, and fashion consumers, *Ms.* redefined women as thinkers, activists, politicians, and citizens deserving of basic human rights.

To launch the magazine, Steinem pitched the founder of *New York* magazine, Clay Felker, on including *Ms.* magazine as a thirty-page insert. The initial run of 300,000 copies sold out in eight days.

In a 1973 interview with the BBC, Steinem said, "It would have been much easier to not start . . . but it was just clear that there was no other way we could be honest about women's experience."

Gloria Steinem wasn't going to just wait for opportunities to present themselves. Instead, she was going to create them herself. As she put it, "Whatever you want to do, just do it."

KEY INSIGHTS

TRADEMARK	Initiating
GIFTS	Having big visions, making the first move
CHALLENGES	Suppressing your urges, waiting for people and opportunities to come to you, taking it personally if your ideas are misunderstood just because they are new, moving forward without keeping others informed
WORK NEEDS	Freedom to act on new ideas, time to recharge alone and work independently, space to stay in your flow without needing to stop and ask for permission at each step, being kept in the loop about any changes that will impact you
RELATIONSHIP NEEDS	Comfort in asking for what you want, support in taking the lead, trust that others will step up when needed, intentional communication that fosters respect and inspires you to share, freedom from being pestered with unwanted questions

This is a perfect example of her Initiate and Inform Strategy as a Manifestor.

At Work

As a Manifestor, you are the only type designed to initiate. You are not meant to wait for anything from the outside world to spur you into action. Rather, you are designed to wait until a desire to take action takes root within you and then to follow that urge. Whether it's pitching a new role, starting a business, reaching out to a collaborator, or disrupting an existing process, you have an innate capacity to create opportunities.

Your ability to take the first step is what sets you apart; this is a gift to embrace, not shy away from. It takes courage to follow your inner impulse to initiate, particularly when walking an untraveled path, but it's how the best things start for you. You might struggle if you're overly passive, waiting for opportunities to come instead of trusting yourself to pursue your visions, or if you shut down the urges that are bubbling up within you. Remember this: Your visions are meant to be pursued and your ideas are meant to become reality, just as Gloria Steinem believed when she created *Ms.* magazine.

While your gift lies in initiating, it's essential to create space for your next inspiration to arrive. One of the best ways to do this is by allowing moments of rest and solitude in your days, because these are often the times when new ideas and impulses naturally surface. Constant busyness can drown out these creative whispers, making it difficult to hear and experience them. When you begin to feel burned out or overwhelmed, try handing off a day-to-day responsibility or taking a day off so you can free your mind for new ideas to emerge.

I met with a Manifestor CEO who perfectly embodied this practice of creating space. She initially came to me feeling uninspired and creatively blocked, unsure of her next steps in the business. She admitted that she knew she worked best by going hard for an intense, inspired burst, followed by a period of solitude to recharge. She *knew* all of this, but she just wasn't doing it in practice. I encouraged her to design a schedule that reflected her optimal way of operating. During her absence in these periods of solitude, her team managed daily operations, which allowed her the space for new ideas to emerge—often during long walks, showers, or even while reading fiction. Once a new burst of inspiration hit, she'd return to her team clear, rejuvenated, and ready to hit the ground running. Allowing herself to rest created the space necessary for her vision and creativity to reemerge, and once again, her business began to thrive.

Similarly, another client who worked in marketing found herself feeling stagnant and dull at work. She decided to take a monthlong sabbatical to reconnect with her inspiration. One month later, she emerged with a fresh approach to client work, pitched it to her boss, and dove right in, her fire reignited.

As a Manifestor, you flourish in work environments where you're free to initiate and act on your ideas. Consider how you can create a work dynamic that supports this. This might look like proposing a new endeavor to your boss or having a discussion with them about how to integrate more flexibility into your schedule, like remote days or fewer meetings. It could also mean talking with your collaborator about allowing yourself time every few weeks to work independently to make space for new inspiration to emerge.

Another essential part of your Strategy is informing, which means keeping those you work with in the loop about your plans and decisions before you set them in motion. Because you are independent, it may be tempting to go off and do things on your own. However, as a Manifestor, your energy and actions are impactful, and your decisions will be felt. By letting your managers, clients, and collaborators know what you're going to do before you do it, you're more likely to gain the support and freedom you need to thrive. Informing helps others feel respected and clears the path for you to do what you're meant to. It is not about seeking permission or justifying your actions; it's simply about giving people a heads-up before you fly. It gives your collaborators a glimpse into your process while you remain firmly in control and in the driver's seat. Though you might initially feel like informing is a hurdle, it's meant to eliminate obstacles and make your col-

laborations more effective and harmonious. For example, say you're leading a project and decide to pivot the strategy based on new insights. By
taking a few minutes to inform your team of the change before executing
it, you not only prevent confusion and resistance, you foster trust and collective alignment. This simple act of communication lets you move forward
with confidence and removes any unnecessary roadblocks.

Make sure to inform others once you've made a decision, but before
taking action. When you share too early, you open yourself to unwanted
feedback. By waiting to share until you're clear, you create space to access answers from within, while ensuring others don't feel disrespected or
excluded from the process. When you inform, you shouldn't be looking for
a specific response or sense of approval from others, or take it personally
when others don't immediately grasp your vision—remember, your strength
lies in seeing things before others do. Think of informing as a practice of
courtesy, not consensus. Also, let people know when you've chosen *not* to
do something they may be expecting you to do. For instance, if you decide
to shut down an offering you've provided your clientele for years, instead
of quietly removing it from your list of services, communicate this change
to current and past customers who will be affected.

Understand that it's not necessary to broadcast your plans to everyone. The idea is to share your decisions with those who will be directly
impacted, not the whole world. One client found that the easiest way to
inform was by scheduling an email or sending a text message, which
allowed him to keep those who needed to be aware in the loop without
him needing to be immediately available for their responses. When not
in a leadership position, it's ideal to establish a dynamic with your boss
where you first align on a vision and direction. Then, you simply keep
them informed on your progress rather than pausing to seek permission
at every step.

Informing should be a two-way street. Not only is it beneficial for you to
keep your collaborators posted about your decisions but it's beneficial for
them to do the same for you. You make others feel respected by informing
them and it is equally important for you to feel respected in return. Also,
Manifestors tend not to enjoy being pestered with unnecessary questions,

so informing and being informed allows you to stay in the know on your own terms without being pulled out of your creative flow.

Your Strategy serves a dual purpose: it empowers you to create the change you desire in your career and ensures ease and respect in your collaborations as you do so. So often, my Manifestor clients have spent their lives sitting on the sidelines, waiting for opportunities to come when *they* are actually meant to be the ones to make the first move. By trusting yourself to initiate and informing others along the way, you clear the path for your visions to come to life.

From Boredom to Trailblazer

Jen had been practicing law for a decade when she came to me. She felt restless and bored, weighed down by performing the same tasks and working with the same clients for years on end.

She loved her firm and she especially loved her vision for how they could be a cutting-edge, pioneering law practice, but she felt bored by her role. She yearned for something new and more inspiring. She couldn't help but see the future, but innovating and restructuring the firm was not in her job description. She dreamed of a scenario where her job wasn't merely about practicing law but advancing it.

"I just can't shake the feeling," Jen confided, her eyes filled with possibility. "I see so much potential for us to lead, to really innovate in law, but my role feels so . . . constrained."

I nodded and smiled. "Well, that makes a lot of sense. You're not meant to follow; you're meant to lead. The cutting edge is exactly where you're supposed to be."

She looked at me hesitantly. "But how? I don't want to leave the firm I love. I'm just so bored of this role."

"That's the beauty of being a Manifestor," I told her. "You are meant to be the one to initiate change, to create the role you dream of. You don't have to wait for permission or for someone to hand you an opportunity."

Inspired, Jen crafted a pitch for a role that didn't exist—a position centered on streamlining operations and enhancing cross-departmental collaboration within the firm. Nervous but determined, she shared the idea with her partners. To her delight, they were on board. They recognized how much she had already improved processes within her existing role and were eager to support her in a new role where she could dedicate herself to optimizing workflows and driving innovation across the firm.

Fast-forward three months, and Jen told me, "I finally found my groove once I felt empowered to create my own role. I'm not just slotting into what has been done before; I'm creating something new." Her smile was contagious; I couldn't help but smile too.

Discovering she was a Manifestor gave Jen permission to approach her career with newfound confidence and creativity. She wasn't just doing her job; she was redefining it as she went, and in doing so, she felt more purposeful and peaceful than ever before.

In Relationships

It's this simple: when you feel the urge to pursue a romantic or platonic connection, follow it. Let the person know what you want and make your intentions clear. This doesn't guarantee success every time—rejection is a part of life, after all—but initiating is the most natural way for you to begin a new relationship. One client shared, "If I hadn't initiated my relationship and informed my now-husband of how I felt, we wouldn't be together now."

Embracing your initiating nature in relationships also means getting comfortable with asking for what you want and sometimes suggesting new or alternative ways of doing things inside a relationship. The fact is, you are not meant to do things the way others do. One client suggested living in a separate apartment from her husband because it felt right even though none of her friends had done it. They've now been happily living separately for ten years. As Gloria Steinem once reflected, "I assumed I had to get married. Everybody did. If you didn't, you were crazy. But I kept putting it off: 'I'm going to do it, but not right now.' Until I was in my late thirties and the women's movement came along, and I realized: I'm happy. Not everyone has to live the same way."

As a Manifestor, you are inherently discerning about people, which can make others less likely to pursue you, so it's more natural for you to break down the barrier and reach out yourself. I can't tell you the number of clients, especially women, who initially felt uncomfortable with the idea of making the first move. Yet when they reflected on their relationships, they realized that the most meaningful ones were those they had initiated, often on a whim.

One Manifestor client was struggling with dating. Her coach advised her to sit back and wait for partners to approach her, but this strategy left her feeling disempowered and like she was bad at dating. When she realized that initiating was the key to her success, she found the courage to ask people out and start the business she'd always dreamed of. Though initiating felt scary, she soon discovered it opened the door to far more promising opportunities.

Initiating a connection doesn't mean you always have to take the lead once the relationship is in place. It's simply how your relationships start best. While it's important to feel free to take the lead and do things your way in a relationship and in a community, once trust is established, it can be nourishing—and even revolutionary—to step back and let others lead every so often. This can be a relief to your nervous system, especially if you're taking charge in other areas of your life. A client in her thirties once shared how liberating it felt to sit in the passenger seat of her car, let her mother take the lead, and simply surrender to the day. She craved occasionally stepping out of a leadership role and handing the reins to those she trusted. Another Manifestor client shared with her partner that, while she might initiate intimacy sometimes, she also enjoyed being pursued.

If you don't feel empowered to lead in your relationships, you may feel dissatisfied and limited. At the same time, you may burn out if you never let others take the lead. Feeling the freedom to lead and *also* trusting others to do so are equally essential ingredients for healthy relationships, whether romantic or platonic.

As with your career, informing those close to you about changes or plans that may affect them is simple yet impactful. Maintaining a strong line of communication helps build trust and prevents misunderstandings and friction. For example, let a new romantic prospect know you'll be offline for a week and will be in touch when you return. Inform your partner if you'll be home late, need time alone, or aren't feeling up for a planned gathering. Your energy is impactful, and people will feel your actions either way; informing simply conveys respect and lets others into your process.

A Manifestor client used to wonder why she had to explain herself when she was just living her life, but she could sense how frazzled and distant her partner became when he learned about the latest work project or a trip she'd already booked. Once she let him in on her decisions, their connection grew stronger and their communication flowed more easily. Be explicit when informing by saying something like, "I'm not looking for your advice right now; I'm simply letting you know because I respect you and our relationship." This reminds others not to disrespect you by questioning or trying to tell you what to do. If you feel controlled or judged, you may communicate less, which no one wants. One client shared that he hesitated to socialize because people always reacted when he slipped out of a gathering; he learned that simply giving people a heads-up let him slip out without guilt and without anyone making a fuss. Another client said, "I used to be afraid of informing because I worried people would get mad, but I've learned that tension only arises when I *don't* inform."

Also, remember that informing should be reciprocal. A Manifestor client shared that she and her Manifestor husband start each day by sharing their plans. This helps them understand each other's schedules, which makes their dynamic more effortless and allows them to offer one another backup when necessary, like making dinner when they see the other has a busy day ahead. She said, "Informing allows us to truly be a team."

Notice the specificity of the word *inform*. For example, instead of your roommate asking what you want for dinner, they could inform you they're ordering in, giving you the option to join if you'd like. Informing you of their evening plans allows you to decide if you want to participate without pressure. Even having someone say, "I'd love to know what you worked on today if you feel inspired to share," allows you to share when you're ready and excited, and on your terms. This approach avoids the annoyance that can arise when someone badgers you with questions and requests and expects an immediate response, allowing you to communicate from a place of genuine inspiration rather than obligation.

So be brave in initiating connections—even if it feels intimidating—and trust that keeping the right people in the loop will only strengthen your relationships.

Making the First Move

Jaclyn often felt the urge to make the first move when dating but, too often, would lose her nerve. She'd spot someone who intrigued her, start walking over, then veer to the bathroom instead at the last minute. Raised to believe men should pursue relationships, she talked herself out of approaching prospective partners time and time again even when she wanted to. And the men who *did* approach Jaclyn were never the ones she was actually drawn to.

By the time she came to me, Jaclyn was feeling disheartened and had reached a point where she felt like romantic relationships were her Achilles' heel. She wanted to be in a relationship but didn't know how to get there.

"Jaclyn, your instinct is right," I confirmed. "You are meant to be the one to pursue relationships. This doesn't mean you have to initiate everything once you're in a relationship, but the best relationships are often the ones you start. This means following those urges you've been ignoring and boldly expressing what you want."

Of course, not every relationship she pursued would succeed, but the first step was having the courage to try.

She laughed knowingly, realizing her impulse had been right. As she thought more about it, she had initiated her most meaningful relationships—with both her ex-boyfriend of five years and her best friend—on the spur of the moment. She had seen her ex-boyfriend across the park and, in a brazen moment of courage, marched up to him and asked him out. On the first day of graduate school, she'd told her soon-to-be best friend she wanted to be friends; they moved in together soon after.

Jaclyn left our session feeling empowered, nervous, and excited about the future. She was relieved to know that waiting for things to happen didn't work for a reason and that there was another way.

The last time we spoke, she told me she had started making the first move more often. While it still scared her and only one pursuit led to a first date so far, it felt exciting, and that first date was the best she'd been on in years. Most importantly, she felt liberated because she was finally embracing what came naturally.

Practices

If you're struggling to find relationships or opportunities that excite you, these practices can help you adopt a new Strategy that, while potentially daunting, can align you with the right people and experiences. If you're already bravely initiating opportunities and feeling at ease in your relationships, these practices will only increase the quality of your connections and experiences.

1. **Consider what you genuinely believe and feel inspired to create.**

   You are here to innovate, to venture where no one has before, and to infuse everything you do with originality and a sense of newness. Whether it's launching a new company, implementing a novel approach within your team or romantic partnership, introducing a way to shake up an industry, or sharing a groundbreaking concept with your community, you inspire people to get on board with your vision when you take action on the ideas that come to you.

Consider where you're holding back from pursuing something new because you don't know how it'll be received. Yes, your ideas may be misunderstood at first or you might not know exactly how they will manifest . . . and that's okay. Regardless of the unknowns—and even of the outcome—treat the visions that come to you as sacred and worth acting on.

2. **Practice initiating in small ways.**

If taking the lead and initiating in your career or life feels intimidating, try starting with small steps to reconnect with your innate power.

Initiating on a smaller scale, such as a hobby you're passionate about, a friendship, or a small collaboration at work, can help build your confidence and gain trust that making the first move will lead to good things. This trust in yourself opens the door to initiate bigger, more significant opportunities.

You may not have been taught to initiate and go after what you want, but as a Manifestor, with time, you will almost certainly discover it's the most effective path toward creating a fulfilling, inspiring career and community. This is not for everyone, but it *is* for you.

3. **Reflect on who will be impacted by your decision before taking action.**

Considering who will be affected by each decision you make is a powerful way to build awareness around the impact of your decisions and actions.

Once you've reflected on who will be impacted, make it a habit to inform them of your decision. This doesn't necessarily have to be a big proclamation or even a conversation; it may look as simple as writing an email, making a call, or sending a text message.

The decision could be as significant as telling a partner you're applying to law school or informing your family you're quitting your job. It might be as small as letting a friend know you won't make it to a gathering or telling a roommate you'll be home late.

While informing might feel cumbersome at first, it's a practice worth honing. It helps deepen trust in your relationships and lets the people that matter into your process.

Journal Prompts

Where do you wish you were braver in your life?

Do you act on the ideas that come to you? What has happened when you have? If not, what's holding you back now?

Do you usually keep people in the loop with your decisions? What do you notice when you do? What happens when you don't?

Do you tend to make the first move in your relationships? What is different when you do? What changes when you don't? How did your most meaningful relationships start?

Who do you trust to take the lead, and how does it feel to step back when they do? Do you wish this happened more often, and why?

Wait a Lunar Cycle

AMMA WAS JUST A YOUNG GIRL WHEN PEOPLE BEGAN MAKING PIL-grimages from around the world to receive her embrace.

Born in a seaside village in Kerala, India, Amma's life took a turn at nine years old when she left school to care for her ailing mother and seven siblings. While collecting food scraps from neighbors, she became acutely aware of the poverty around her and started sharing whatever she could from her own home. During these visits, neighbors would confide in her, and moved by their pain, Amma began embracing them, finding it the most natural way to offer comfort. As she explains, "This is my inborn nature. The duty of a doctor is to treat patients. In the same way, my duty is to console those who are suffering."

What began as a simple act of kindness grew into something much larger, though Amma never intended to create a global movement. As word spread, people began calling her Amma, which means "mother" in Sanskrit, and traveled long distances for her embrace. Brief moments in her arms were described as "a big, rapturous hug . . . an infusion of pure, unconditional love" in *Rolling Stone*. Some even moved into her family home, becoming her disciples, and invitations soon poured in for her to share her hugs abroad.

KEY INSIGHTS

TRADEMARK	Sensitivity to your environment
GIFTS	Finding the best opportunities and relationships by being in spaces that feel right, tapping into your sensitivity to attract opportunities
CHALLENGES	Spending time in workspaces or with people who sap your energy, keeping to yourself in new settings, chasing opportunities instead of letting the right ones find you, settling for situations where your gifts go unnoticed
WORK NEEDS	Trusting that your perspective makes a difference, having your needs considered, working with people and in spaces that put you at ease
RELATIONSHIP NEEDS	Respect for your sensitivity to your surroundings, invitations to share your thoughts, thought-provoking questions, facilitation of new opportunities, curiosity about how you operate best

Today Amma has traveled the world and embraced over forty million people. Her humanitarian work in India has led to the creation of hospitals, universities, and countless initiatives to alleviate suffering.

Amma's ability to let opportunities arise naturally without chasing or forcing them perfectly reflects her Strategy of Wait a Lunar Cycle as a Reflector.

At Work

In Human Design, the Strategy for Reflectors is often presented as Wait a Lunar Cycle, and their Strategy and Authority are collapsed into one concept. While it is essential for Reflectors to be patient and wait twenty-eight to thirty days when making decisions (more on this soon), they can use additional tools to create opportunities that often get skipped over. With this in mind, I want to introduce a new take on the Reflector Strategy to add color to how you can be proactive in creating career opportunities.

As a Reflector, your acuity and perspective are truly unique gifts. You possess the ability to understand issues from various angles and to offer clear, unbiased insights on how and where things could be improved. Reflectors are invaluable for their capacity to inspire change in spaces, communities, or teams. Often, just a single Reflector can catalyze transformation. This is why they're so rare.

To ensure your wisdom will be valued in your work environment, it's best to share your insights when you're specifically invited or welcomed to do so, like Projectors. Put simply, you shine at work when your perspective is sought after, and you are encouraged to share all that you see. You want to reserve your valuable, objective wisdom for those who are genuinely receptive and ready to appreciate it, where it can have the most profound impact. Ideal collaborators will not only welcome your vision but are eager to implement your suggestions when they're useful and can make a difference.

Challenge or burnout may arise if you chase recognition and opportunities instead of allowing the right people to discover your unique talents, or if you settle for opportunities where your rare gifts are overlooked or undervalued. It's a sign of a potential mismatch when a collaborator doesn't understand your approach and pressures you to do things the way everyone else is doing them. Being understood—or at least having the people you work with make a concerted effort to understand you—is a key indicator of a promising collaboration. Acknowledgment of the usefulness and originality of your viewpoint ensures that your gifts and way of working are respected, sparing you from the pressure to conform or constantly produce.

When it comes to communication in a work environment, in addition to waiting to share until you feel your perspective is valued, it can help to clearly express your own needs and desires, especially given that they may differ from those of your colleagues. Remember, your gifts are exceptional and impactful, and the right collaborators will see and value that.

As a Reflector, the most effective way to attract career opportunities is to place yourself in environments that resonate with you. You've likely heard the quote from motivational speaker Jim Rohn: "You're the average of the five people you spend the most time with." While some nuance is lost when we look only at the five people around us, a kernel of truth exists in these words: we are heavily influenced by the people and places we choose. And there's no other type that this is truer for than Reflectors. This means choosing the right city, office, and/or co-working space is not a "nice to have"; it's essential. When asked how they gauge whether or not a space feels right, the most common response from Reflectors was that they felt a sense of ease, belonging, presence, and possibility. Comfortable environments and spaces will naturally lead to opportunities, experiences, and invitations aligned with your path. The more you prioritize being in energetically aligned spaces and stepping away from those that are not, the smoother your career will flow.

In practice, this can mean checking out the office of a potential job to see if it resonates with you or immersing yourself in environments—both online and in the real world—that are inspiring when you feel stuck, like a café or workspace you love, or an online community that motivates you. Or it could mean choosing the restaurant to meet a potential collaborator at, knowing the best connections happen in settings that feel comfortable. Only you can determine what feels right, but you will recognize these places when you find them. You may also find a space feels uplifting and energizing for a period of time, and then stops feeling that way. As one client shared, "Sometimes, the same place at the wrong time does not feel friendly, easy, and available, and I won't feel like I belong there. Timing is everything."

A Reflector client shared that she had never landed a job through a traditional application. Instead, her opportunities always arose from serendipitous connections. For instance, while working as a waitress at a wine bar, she met a patron who asked about her aspirations. When she mentioned her dream of working for the United Nations, the woman offered her a job on the spot at the nongovernmental organization she led, which was headquartered at the UN and where my client spent the next seven years. Later, she attended a grant-writing workshop she was excited about. The instructor hired her immediately, and she pivoted into a freelance grant writing career for three years. Each opportunity came unexpectedly, flowing naturally from being in the right place at the right time. As she explained, "I shine in spaces where people are both interested and interesting, where I feel I'm being received, and where something I've said piques their curiosity—often surprising even me. My power lies in showing others who I am and what I can do, not in convincing them to give me a chance." This serves as a powerful reminder for Reflectors: simply being in the right space with the right people and showing up authentically can open the door to unexpected opportunities.

To understand the importance of your surroundings, remember that, as a Reflector, you mirror the energy around you. If you're surrounded by creative, motivated entrepreneurs, their drive and inspiration will likely rub off on you, spurring you to chase new ideas too. Conversely, being around those who are disenchanted and unmotivated by their work can dampen your spirit and curb your drive. So, when considering your work environment or opening yourself to new opportunities, focus on the energy that resonates with your aspirations and surround yourself with people who inspire growth in that direction. If you're drawn to art, mingle with artists. If entrepreneurship sparks your interest, connect with fellow entrepreneurs. In short, use your sensitivity as a way to bring new, more fitting opportunities your way.

One client, a coach, was about to launch a new offering. In preparation, she surrounded herself with motivated peers and friends who had successful launches. By curating the energy around her, she achieved her most successful launch yet.

The opposite is also true. Another client felt stagnant in her career and realized during our session that her partner was also feeling stuck. She was mirroring his stagnation in her own life. Once she began working outside the home and exploring new environments, doors began to open.

Being in the right space around the right people is one of the most powerful tools at your disposal to attract the right prospects, connections, and experiences. Once you're in a space that feels expansive with people who feel resonant, stay open to new opportunities and directions as they present themselves, allowing your career to unfold in unforeseen yet fulfilling ways.

The Best Surprise

Mila came to me because she was feeling eager for something new in her career. She had successfully managed a marketing agency for three years. While this role was gratifying at times, it didn't change the fact that it no longer felt right to her. She felt a desire to go after and create something new but didn't have a clue what that next thing was, and it was stressing her out. The need for change was clear but the direction was not.

"Should I already know what's next?" she asked, worry etched into every line on her face.

"Not at all," I reassured her. "The best opportunities appear when you're in the right environment and surrounded by the right people. Sometimes, you won't recognize these moments until they happen."

Mila laughed as she began to recall how all of her past career opportunities had spontaneously emerged. Her journey into launching an agency had begun by chance over coffee at her favorite café. Impressed by Mila's marketing chops, a former colleague she admired had encouraged her to strike out on her own. So, she did. Successfully. Her corporate role prior to that had also started unexpectedly in a coworking space, where a casual conversation with another member led to an incredible job offer.

Reflecting on her career, Mila realized that all of the most fulfilling opportunities had appeared not through active pursuit but simply by spending time in spaces she enjoyed with people she felt inspired by.

"This pattern . . . it's *always* been about where I am and who I'm with," she mused. I could sense Mila's relief that her next steps suddenly felt accessible.

After our session, Mila reached out to beloved clients and collaborators for coffee chats at her favorite spots. She entered into those conversations open to discovering what might come next. In one of those meetings, the next steps were illuminated (as they always had been) when a former client expressed admiration for Mila's writing. "I've always loved the way you write. Would you consider editing my book manuscript?" the client proposed.

Though it diverged from her expectations, Mila was thrilled by the prospect of this new path. It seemed like a surprising yet perfect blend of new challenges and her existing skill set.

And just like that, Mila embarked on the next chapter of her career.

In Relationships

You may feel disappointed in how few new meaningful relationships arrive in your life if you don't make an effort to spend time in spaces that you genuinely enjoy. As with your career, the best relationships emerge when you invest time in online and offline places that nourish and invigorate you at once. For example, you might strike up a rich conversation with a stranger that turns into a deep friendship at your favorite coffee shop or meet a collaborator at a conference you're excited to attend.

You attract aligned relationships when you are open and present in these environments, ready for anything that comes your way. Whereas, you might have a hard time if you enter into new spaces and keep to yourself rather than remaining curious about whatever (and whoever) awaits you there. In a moment of unexpected delight at her favorite vacation spot, a happily single client of mine met her now-husband. One Reflector said, "One of my favorite things is to go out alone. I love seeing who life will bring me. Often, I'm invited into a new dynamic when I'm in my favorite spaces, whether it's a friend group, an interesting conversation, or a flirtation." Another client shared how her most meaningful relationships came to life. She met one friend when they randomly sat next to each other and felt an immediate connection at a coaching school. Another friendship blossomed through a shared sports club; the spark was instant when the stranger approached her. She also felt an instantaneous bond and made a dear friend in a Facebook group for a mutual hobby; the minute they started talking, they felt as if they'd known each other for years. Her now-boyfriend appeared at her favorite club, and their chemistry was immediate too. She shared, "I didn't initiate the connections; I simply chose to be in a space I enjoyed, and the rest just happened." She also shared that, despite understanding the power of comfortable spaces, she never enters them with the expectation of connection and is always genuinely surprised when they manifest as they do.

It's important to show up as yourself when you meet new people and notice the relationships where the connection comes easily and brings out a version of yourself that you love, which is easiest while in comfortable spaces. While new acquaintances may not immediately recognize everything about you—that would be impossible—you *should* feel an invitation to share yourself freely. This is a sign a relationship is worth exploring.

You may struggle if you have low standards and jump in with anyone who shows up rather than taking the time to assess whether you feel sincere curiosity from that person. Sincere curiosity can look like someone asking meaningful questions and demonstrating an interest in your unique perspective on the world.

As a Reflector, it's important to continue honoring your sensitivity to your environment as you explore new relationships and deepen existing ones. If a café doesn't feel right for a date, suggest a last-minute change to another that does, or make it a practice of selecting the restaurant yourself. If you're on a friend date and find you don't like the vibes at a table or venue, switch without guilt or a second thought.

You are most supported in relationships when words of affirmation are offered often, you are asked thoughtful questions, and you feel free to share whatever version of yourself feels most true in the moment. Feeling continually invited to share yourself throughout your many evolutions and having your perspective cherished are integral to a healthy, lasting relationship. It may also delight you when loved ones initiate you into new opportunities and relationships, as friends who know you well can be invaluable in guiding you toward the right next step in your life.

Right Space, Good Life

Sara had been trying dating apps for months without success. She was feeling discouraged that she'd had no success up to this point, unlike many of her friends who'd found partners online.

I could hear the note of hopelessness in her voice as she asked if she should keep trying. "Is it just a matter of timing, or should I give up?" Often, we lose hope not because something is impossible, but because we're taking the wrong approach. This is exactly what was happening for Sara.

"Sara," I said, "it seems the approach you're using may not be right for you. The right relationships—romantic or otherwise—will come when you're in a space you love. This space can even be online—though, based on our conversation, it doesn't sound like apps are that place for you."

I suggested that Sara delete the apps for now and instead explore planting herself in spaces that resonated with her, remaining open to whatever came her way in the process.

She smiled and nodded. While she wasn't fully convinced this approach would work, it sounded more enjoyable than what she'd been doing.

Sara's first step was to return to her favorite salsa class at a local dance studio, a place that had always brought her joy. At first, nothing seemed to shift except for the fact that she was far happier because she was dancing more and spending time in one of her favorite places. In addition, she started working from cozy, plant-filled cafés, took leisurely walks with friends through beautiful parks, and made a point of rediscovering the joys of her neighborhood in a way she hadn't since first moving there.

Just a few weeks after adopting this strategy, someone she'd been eyeing at the dance studio asked her out. The scenario felt effortless and natural, and Sara felt excited and open, so she said yes.

Though the relationship was still new, Sara felt a profound sense of relief after stepping away from the draining online spaces that had once consumed her. She embraced the belief that spending time in environments she truly enjoys was the key to attracting meaningful relationships and experiences. This approach felt more empowering and easeful than any she had tried before.

Practices

If you're struggling to find opportunities and relationships that bring out your best, these practices can help draw more aligned ones your way. If you're already fulfilled by how you're spending your time and who you're spending it with, these practices will help you stay on course and smoothly adapt to changes as they come.

1. **Begin to notice your sensitivity to space.**

    Pay attention to how a space feels in your body. Ask yourself if a space makes you feel open, relaxed, at ease, and inspired, or tense, closed off, and uncomfortable.

    Trust the wisdom of your body to guide you exactly where you need to go. You may find that many of your most meaningful interactions emerge in unpredictable ways, and in spaces you love. Create more opportunities for these moments. Visit your favorite spots alone and notice who shows up and makes you feel treasured. Be open to surprise. And remember that it's okay to leave spaces that don't feel right even if they once did.

2. **Pay attention to what it feels like to be genuinely recognized when you are out in a new space.**

    Identify what makes you feel seen when meeting someone new and notice how it feels in your body when an authentic connection is sparked. Let that list be a blueprint for you going forward.

    You might even want to look back at how you connected with your favorite people and opportunities. Often, reflecting on how your most successful, surprising, and delightful relationships and experiences came to life can offer insight into what to look out for going forward. Our past offers clues if we take the time to listen.

3. **Consider the energy you wish to magnify in your life.**

    As someone who naturally reflects your surroundings, choose what you mirror with purpose. What aspects do you want to embody more in your life? Is it about connecting with those who balance parenting alongside their careers? Or immersing yourself in the company of entrepreneurs who value both time and financial freedom? Perhaps it's drawing inspiration from creatives who express themselves boldly

How Do You Choose?

through their work or refining your speaking skills alongside seasoned professionals in the field.

Whatever the thing is for you, identify the energy that resonates alongside it and seek out environments and individuals who embody these qualities. By doing so, those qualities will come alive within you.

Journal Prompts

Which spaces feel best to you right now, and why?

Where is your perspective sought after and most impactful at work? If your perspective is recognized in this way, how does it feel? If not, do you desire this?

What type of energy do you wish to invite into your life? Is it the creative, inspiring energy of artists, the resourceful, vitalizing energy of entrepreneurs, or something else altogether? Why?

How did your most meaningful relationships start? Do you see any patterns?

Who honors your sensitivity to space? How does it feel when this is respected? If it is not, how could you better express this need to friends?

3

Authority

How You Make Decisions

- Your Authority reveals how to assess which opportunities and relationships are right for you.

- It offers insights about how to tap into your intuition, how to choose the best opportunities and relationships, how to get out of your head, how to keep the faith even when others disagree, and how to communicate your decision-making process to those you love.

- There are seven Authorities: Sacral, Emotional, Splenic, Self-Projected, Ego, Mental, and None.

KEY INSIGHTS

PERCENT OF POPULATION	35
TRADEMARK	A strong gut feeling
LOOK FOR	The visceral feeling in your belly before your mind has a chance to get in the way, whether your body pulls you toward or pushes you away from an opportunity, the natural enthusiasm or hesitation in your voice
GIFTS	Instantly knowing if someone or something is right
CHALLENGES	Trying to rationalize your gut feeling and ultimately talking yourself out of it, delaying decisions instead of trusting your immediate knowing, ignoring your gut because of the uncertainty about the outcome, feeling swallowed up by others' feelings about a decision
RELATIONSHIP NEEDS	Respect for your gut instinct without needing to explain it, freedom to make quick decisions and change your mind, space to be alone and reconnect with your gut instinct when needed

Sacral

IN THE MUSIC BUSINESS, THERE IS A TIME-TESTED WAY TO LAUNCH A record. Typically, this begins with teaser campaigns on social media, followed by the release of a lead single and music video. Preorders and exclusive merchandise are often made available to fans alongside strategic partnerships with streaming services for playlist placements. Finally, the record is launched with a series of live performances, such as a release concert or tour to maximize exposure and drive sales.

On the morning of December 13, 2013, Beyoncé fans around the world discovered that their precious Bey didn't need to do any of that to capture their imaginations. Without warning, her fifth studio album was available for purchase. No marketing necessary. Additionally, she required fans to purchase the entire album instead of being able to stream individual songs, a daring decision in an era dominated by singles.

In a press release accompanying the album's launch, she explained, "I didn't want to release the music the way I've done it. I am bored with that . . . I just want this to come out when it's ready and from me to my fans."

The album's success was unprecedented. It became the fastest-selling album on iTunes at the time, reached number one in over one hundred countries, and won three Grammy Awards.

By following her gut instinct in the face of the status quo, Beyoncé shows us what it means to live with a Sacral Authority.

How Do You Choose?

At Work

When an opportunity comes your way, you are meant to make a decision in the moment based on your gut feeling, an unmistakable, visceral response to what's in front of you. It's a certainty in your belly that either draws you in or pushes you away. Unlike many, you have the capacity for instant clarity, and this applies to big and small decisions alike. As soon as you feel a full-bodied yes in your gut, you're meant to follow and act on that instinct, even if you don't know where it will take you. If you receive anything less than a full-bodied yes, it either means the opportunity isn't right, or the timing is off, even if the *no* doesn't feel strong or loud.

A yes in your gut may feel like an excited buzz, a sense of internal expansion, a rising of energy, an unshakeable certainty, a feeling of happiness devoid of any anxiety or doubt, an open and calm sensation in your stomach, a feeling that your body is being pulled toward an opportunity, or a note of eagerness in your voice.

A no may appear as an uncomfortable knot, a sigh, a heaviness, a contraction in your belly, a sense of discomfort when thinking about the opportunity, or a hitch in your voice. It might feel like your energy is recoiling or being pulled away. You might find yourself feeling drained at just the thought of the opportunity. Or you may simply feel nothing at all.

Your gut feeling is not just a tool for determining where to put your energy; it also tells you *when* to do so. An opportunity may not feel right when it's initially presented but a week (or year) later, it could. My husband has this Authority and uses a "now-or-not-now" framework when making decisions. If he feels excited by both the opportunity and the timing, he treats it as a *now*, commits fully, and acts in the moment. If it's anything but that, he waits for his gut feeling to indicate when the timing is right. Sometimes, exciting ideas become *nows* years down the line. One client was invited to a professional development weekend workshop. Even though it seemed useful, and he couldn't identify *why* he shouldn't do it, his body gave him a clear no. Instead of questioning it, he told the organizer it wasn't the right time for him. A month later, the same workshop felt right, so he attended, and there, he met his future business partner.

Here's the hard part about this Authority: your gut feeling does not come with a reason. This means that if you notice yourself trying to rationalize decisions—whether it's taking a job, attending an event, launching a business, or any other career move—you've likely disconnected from your gut. Your gut instinct is simply a feeling that something is right or not—and that feeling comes before logic has had a chance to intervene. If you find yourself saying, "I think I should do this because . . . ," pause and drop into your belly instead, noticing whether you feel expansion or contraction.

Here's the second challenge: your mind won't stop getting in the way. Often, clients have an immediate gut response to an opportunity, only to second-guess it—even when past decisions based on their gut have proven successful. Catch yourself in these moments when you're allowing the endless questioning of your mind to complicate what could be a simple decision. Overthinking makes you feel indecisive when you often already know the answer and are simply struggling to trust it. Decision-making can and should be simple. One client consistently had a gut instinct about new hires but, for years, talked herself out of it. It was only later, when certain hires didn't work out, that she understood why her gut had pointed her elsewhere. Over time, she learned to trust her first instinct, and her team did too.

If you feel excitement in response to a potentiality, but it doesn't feel full-bodied or complete yet, go to the office where you'd be working, meet the colleagues you'd be collaborating with, or do a sample project to see how it feels. Or have someone ask you yes-or-no questions about the opportunity to see if it elicits a clearer response. This deeper engagement will provide a richer experience for your gut to respond to and will help you determine if an opportunity and the timing are truly aligned. Waiting for that full-bodied yes might feel annoying at times, but it's crucial. It ensures you say yes to work commitments you can genuinely sustain and show up for rather than committing to a project only for your energy to wane quickly because it was never right for you in the first place.

With Sacral Authority, it is also important to note you can be easily swayed by the enthusiasm of others. Many clients have shared how they often get so wrapped up in others' feelings about a decision that they lose touch with their own instincts. It is not until they step away from a conversation that they realize their gut is pointing them in a very clear direction that just so happens to differ from the opinion of others. Creating space for yourself after interacting with others can help you reconnect with your instinct and clear away the influence of their excitement or lack thereof. Consider others' advice simply as something to respond to: Does a person's recommendation feel right in your gut or not?

One client organized a group interview session, bringing all potential candidates for a job together to observe their interactions. After the session, he asked two of his employees for their opinion. They both preferred the candidates with the most education and experience; candidates who, in my client's view, were somewhat lackluster and dry. Instead, my client found himself drawn to a younger, less experienced candidate. Despite his employees' skepticism about choosing someone who was less impressive on paper, he trusted his gut instinct, listened to the fact that his employees' advice did not feel right, and hired the candidate who stood out to him. Not only did this hire stay with the company long after the employees my client consulted with left, but he continued to work with my client on subsequent projects after the business ultimately shut down.

Trust that your gut is meant to alert you to the next most-aligned decision in your career without revealing the entire journey. This can be challenging if you value predictability and a ten-year plan. But your path is about making one right decision at a time, trusting that the aggregate of right choices will lead you in the best direction, even if it's different from what you first envisioned. As author and artist Julia Cameron wisely said, "When we are on the right path, we have a surefootedness. We know the next right action—although not necessarily what is just around the bend. By trusting, we learn to trust."

Dream Job Dilemma

David came to me feeling perplexed. Based on his sun-kissed face and the ocean view I could see peeking through his window in the background of our Zoom call, I wasn't surprised to hear that David's career centered around surfing. He explained to me that it had long been his favorite pastime, so straight out of high school, he'd sought a sales position at his surfboard company of choice. When he landed the job, David was convinced he'd found his dream job right out of the gate. Still, he found that he felt oddly indifferent when the job offer came. He dismissed his lack of enthusiasm as normal, but as he settled into the role, the excitement David anticipated never arrived. Despite the fact that the job ticked all the boxes he thought he wanted checked—sharing the sport he loved with others, predictable hours, and good pay—after only a month, David found himself feeling disengaged and bored. Despite this, he pressed on, and by the time we connected, he'd been in the same position for three years.

"How can I be unhappy at my dream job?" he asked me. "I thought this was just the beginning of a long career selling surfboards. I planned on climbing the ranks and settling in, but I'm just so bored."

"According to your Human Design, you are meant to make decisions based on your gut instinct in the moment," I told David gently. "The right opportunities should feel expansive, exciting, and like you can't help but move toward them. Whereas the wrong ones feel deflating, uncomfortable, or leave you feeling indifferent."

I watched as a lightbulb went off for David, and he realized he'd based his career choice on what he *believed* he should want rather than what actually resonated with his gut instinct. Although he loved surfing, selling surfing equipment had never felt right if David was being honest with himself.

Soon after our session, he quit the sales job and decided to pay attention to what felt right in his gut rather than what made sense.

> This led David to discover a new product in a field he never envisioned himself in—technology—and that he continues to be excited about two years later.
>
> And, of course, he still surfs every day.
>
> Sometimes, your gut feeling can take you in unexpected directions . . . and for those with a Sacral Authority, that direction is the right one.

In Relationships

Though it might be tempting to justify why you should or should not pursue a certain relationship, there's a deeper knowing within you—your gut instinct—that serves as an unfailing guide, just like in your career. Unlike others who need time to process, you will quickly feel a strong, gut-level certainty about whether someone is right for you, and that sense will arrive without reason.

When someone is right for you, you'll likely feel an immediate draw toward them, as if your body is being pulled in their direction. This may manifest as a warm, energized feeling, or you might find that your entire being lights up and expands in their presence. They might not fit the image you had in mind in terms of age, career, appearance, or demeanor, yet there is something that just feels true and makes you want to be with and around them. You are not forcing the feeling; it's undeniably there. One client described the sensation as a magnet pulling her toward her now-husband the moment he walked into the restaurant where she worked. Another client's partner with Sacral Authority threw out his wool peacoat upon learning she was allergic to wool the very first night they met because he sensed he'd just met his life partner. And yet another client hadn't even met her partner but felt a deep sense of certainty that he was the one when a mutual friend spoke about him. And, indeed, he was. However it appears, you are designed to trust the immediate feeling in your core.

Trusting your gut instinct applies to all relationships, not just romantic ones. Someone might fit well into your social circle but doesn't feel right for a closer relationship. Or you might feel a gut instinct to explore a relationship without knowing if it will lead to romance or friendship. One client felt an immediate connection with her now-husband and nurtured a yearslong friendship, never seeing him as a romantic partner—until one day, he walked into a party, and she just knew he was the one.

On the other hand, you may experience an immediate sense of contraction when someone who isn't right for you enters your life. Your body might feel like it's pulling away, accompanied by a sinking feeling or sense of unease. You may instinctively want to create space and feel more exhausted after spending time with them. There will be an indefinable (yet physical) sense that something is off. If this happens, it's not necessarily that the person you're reacting to isn't a good person, just that they're not the *right* person for you. One client shared that she often dated people who felt like an immediate no, but they persisted and wore her down until she said yes. She eventually understood why each of them wasn't the correct fit and now realizes that she didn't need to walk those paths when she instinctively knew from the start they weren't a match.

Years ago, a client went on a first date with a man who seemed perfect on paper, checking all her boxes. During the date, he made an offhand comment about disliking ketchup. Though she didn't care much about ketchup herself, her gut instinct immediately told her, "I don't think a partnership with this man would feel dynamic." Ignoring that feeling, she dated him for two years before ultimately realizing it was not the relationship she wanted or needed. She reflected, "I do wonder how my life might have sent me down a different path had I trusted my gut more implicitly back then."

Recently, she went on another first date with a man who also seemed ideal. They had a great time, and the conversation flowed effortlessly. Yet, throughout the evening, a subtle gut feeling kept surfacing: "He's a great guy, but not for me." This time, it took her only two days to listen to that instinct and end things. In her words, "It feels incredible to now trust my gut feeling so powerfully, immediately, and implicitly."

It can be hard at first to trust the feeling that someone isn't right when they seem perfect in every other way and your feeling isn't accompanied by a reason. Yet your gut instinct's purpose is simply to tell you if a relationship is worth pursuing with the reason revealing itself later. One client met a woman at an airport and instantly felt she was the one. The first few years were difficult because they lived in different cities, and his friends urged him to end what they saw as an impractical relationship. Nonetheless, he trusted his instinct and stayed with her. Eventually, they moved in together and got married. Despite knowing she was right for him from the start, it took self-trust to persist when others didn't support his choice.

Your task is to live from the inside out and build enough faith to follow your instinct about people. This also means listening to your gut when it stops saying yes to a relationship. It may have been right once upon a time but simply isn't anymore. One client shared that her partner said something that gave her a sinking feeling. In that moment, she knew he wasn't right for her anymore. Someone can be right for you for a period of time but not necessarily for *all* time. When clients express persistent doubts about their relationship, I ask, "Does this still feel like the right relationship for you?" Often, the immediate, visceral response from the gut is no. (Trusting and acting on this feeling is another story, but the answer is clear.) As with your career, the gut often gives a quick, definite answer when asked a specific yes-or-no question.

You tend to feel most supported in a relationship when others respect your gut instinct and encourage you to trust it without requiring an explanation. You do not feel wrong for making quick decisions or wanting the first thing you see without considering all of your other potential options. There's no pressure to give the expected answer; those who love you want to know what you genuinely feel in your gut. They ask questions without suggesting what they think you should do and offer feedback only if you ask for it. You are given grace for changing your mind when something shifts from a yes to a no or a "not right now."

They may even point out when you don't seem enthusiastic about something or if you come alive talking about something else; they are listening not only to the words you say but also are picking up on your conviction in your gut. One client takes an "I don't know" response from her daughter with Sacral Authority as a no and saves room for a "Heck yes" later down the line. She can always tell when her daughter feels that *yes!* because she can see her daughter's whole body light up. Another client noticed his partner would lean back and shake her head when she was overthinking and lean in with conviction when her gut was leading a conversation.

Once, my partner and I were looking for an Airbnb in the woods to ring in the New Year. I spent weeks researching and found what I thought were excellent options, but he kept saying no to every choice I showed him. Finally, I found a listing with stunning photos but no reviews (never a good sign). I showed it to him, and he immediately said yes, so we booked the place on the spot. That's how the gut instinct works in a nutshell—it's in-the-moment clarity that doesn't need space or time to settle. The house turned out to be perfect, and in fact, we loved it so much that we even asked if it was for sale. It wasn't, but it opened our minds to the possibility of leaving New York City and ultimately kickstarted our move. As we were looking for homes, I fell in love with one that he instantly knew wasn't right. Wanting to support me, he went along with it, doing whatever he could to make it happen even though his gut was screaming no. One night I walked into his room and found him close to tears because he was so overwhelmed by the pressure I was putting on him to go against his gut. This was a big lesson for me as a partner. Needless to say, we did not buy that house, but our dream home appeared soon after. It was an immediate yes for him before we even went inside. Our agent laughed at his enthusiastic response and asked if we had any interest in seeing the actual interior of the house. To this day, we are happily settled in that home in the woods.

It's easy to experience conflict and misunderstanding in a relationship simply because we don't understand how another makes decisions and assume we are wired the same way. While it's important to know our own Authority, it's equally important to understand the Authority of those close to us. This way, we can make decisions that feel right for everyone involved.

The lesson about interacting with a loved one with Sacral Authority was reinforced years later when I spoke with a client who had moved forward with renting a house his girlfriend loved even though it didn't feel right in his gut. The deal was enticing, so my client talked himself out of his gut response, and they moved in. Soon after, he got mold poisoning, and it took him a year to recover.

Sometimes, it can feel difficult to trust your own gut over others' clarity about a relationship or an important choice. Hard as it is, always ensure you're choosing from your gut, not someone else's excitement or disinterest. This might mean taking space, having a third party ask you yes-or-no questions, or investing in a practice that helps you tune into your belly before committing to a relationship or making a big decision. Despite how loud your mind can be, your gut instinct is the voice to listen to when deciding who to let into your life and how to navigate those relationships.

Wedding Woes

Lauren's wedding was three weeks away when we sat down for her session.

"People generally come to me when they're looking for clarity around three areas," I explained. "Relationships, career, and self-care. Is anything coming up for you there?"

"Relationships, for sure," Lauren replied without hesitation.

As I reviewed Lauren's Human Design chart, one piece jumped out at me immediately. Her design revealed that she had a strong gut feeling about the relationships that were right for her and was meant to follow that instinct in the moment—even when it didn't seem to make logical sense.

As I shared this, Lauren began to sob.

"It's the wedding," she said. "It's wrong."

Everything about Lauren's partner seemed perfect in theory. They'd been together for three years. They were great friends. But she wasn't sure if this was it—and if she was being honest with herself, she'd never been sure. Furthermore, both the relationship itself and a planned move across the country after the wedding disrupted her plans to go to medical school to pursue her dream of becoming a dermatologist.

"I love him so much," Lauren said through her tears. "But I feel more trapped and frightened each day as the wedding gets closer. I don't know how to stop the train."

Clearly, Lauren's gut was letting her know that the relationship wasn't fully aligned, but choosing to walk away seemed almost impossible. How often in life do we find ourselves at a crossroads like this? Confronted with a big decision, we grapple with conflicting feelings that ultimately leave us in a perpetual state of indecision. Or worse, we choose a path we already know is wrong.

I sat with Lauren quietly. I'd witnessed this moment of difficult—even painful—clarity thousands of times before in my client sessions, and I know how heart-wrenching it is. After a few moments, I asked her one more question: "Lauren, when did you know he wasn't right for you?"

"From the minute I entered the relationship," she answered quietly.

So often, we know what's right for us and yet still struggle to trust it. We overlook an initial instinct only to realize later—be it days, weeks, months, or years down the line—that we knew the truth from the start.

The most powerful way for Lauren to access her gut feeling was to be asked simple, specific yes-or-no questions and to then pay attention to her immediate gut response—the one that comes before her mind has a chance to jump in and make a case.

"Does this relationship feel right in your gut?" I asked.

Her answer was immediate. "No."

"Lauren, do you want to call off the wedding?"

She responded with a definitive, resounding, albeit somber, "Yes."

Lauren needed permission to trust herself. And in that moment, Human Design gave her all the permission she needed.

Ultimately, Lauren called off the wedding and reenrolled in school. It wasn't easy. But it was easier than living a life that wasn't meant for her. A single powerful but challenging choice shifted Lauren's life from one of frustration and confusion to one of alignment, clarity, and purpose.

Practices

If you feel disconnected from your gut instinct and rarely trust it in your professional or personal life, the following practices will help you build a stronger connection to and confidence in its wisdom. And if you're already in full trust of your gut instinct in all areas of life, big and small, these practices will help maintain and fortify that trust.

1. **Invest your energy in practices that help you connect to your body.**

   Because your gut instinct is belly-based, it helps to invest your energy in any practice that allows you to drop out of your head and into the far more subtle sensations of your belly. Whether it's breathwork, dance, yoga, or any form of embodied practice, the aim is to cultivate a deeper connection with your body and, thus, your gut feeling.

   Then, whenever a person or opportunity shows up, practice dropping into that belly space and paying attention to whether you feel a sense of expansion or contraction, subtle though it may be. Do you feel an inexplicable pull? Or do you shrink and contract? Do you feel ease or discomfort in your belly?

2. **Notice how your gut instinct manifests.**

   The gut feeling can show up differently from one person to the next. Sometimes, it can present vocally as something like an automatic "uh-huh" if it's a yes or an "uh-unh" if it's a no. It may feel like a physical sensation in your belly, perhaps a sense of expansion if it's a yes or discomfort if it's a no. Or it may feel like being pulled toward an opportunity if it's a yes or pushed away if it's a no.

   The list goes on, but these responses all have one thing in common: they arise as feelings or sensations, not as logic or reason. Pay attention to and notice what your own yes and no responses feel like. The more familiar you become with these sensations, the easier and more natural your decisions will be.

3. **Have a conversation with someone close to you about the importance of your gut feeling in your decisions.**

    Human Design teaches us that we all make decisions differently. While your gut instinct is a reliable guide, others have their own process for connecting to their knowing.

    With this in mind, have a conversation with someone close to you about the role of your gut instinct in decision-making. Explain to them that your gut feeling doesn't come with a reason. Let them know that your clarity comes in the moment, not over time. Share with them how they can help you connect with your gut instincts, like asking you specific yes-or-no questions or paying attention to your body's visceral response when they suggest something.

    Set them up to support you in leading from your gut, and learn more about how they make decisions so you can support them in leading from their own knowing too.

Journal Prompts

Do you feel connected to your gut feeling? If so, what sensations signal a yes for you, and which ones indicate a no?

When choosing new work opportunities, do you trust your gut or rely on logic? Which works better for you, and why?

Have any recent opportunities felt right in your gut? If so, are you pursuing them? If not, what's holding you back?

Who respects your gut instinct without needing an explanation? How does that feel, and do you want more of it?

In which relationships do you feel free to make quick decisions? Where do you feel pressured to slow down and think it over? Which approach feels better, and why?

Emotional

IN 2008 AS GLOBAL MARKETS CRUMBLED AND THE US FACED ITS worst economic crisis since the 1930s, the collapse of one of the largest investment banks, Lehman Brothers, sent the financial world into a panic. Senior equity trader Ryan Larson told the *New York Times* that September, "You just felt like the world was unraveling. . . . People started to sell and they sold hard. It didn't matter what you had—you sold."

Amid the chaos, Warren Buffett, one of the most successful investors of the twentieth century, remained composed. While others reacted emotionally and rushed to sell off assets, Buffett did not allow himself to be rattled by the chaos. He continued to make decisions in the way he always did: calmly and patiently.

Instead of selling, Buffett bought. He invested in American stocks and companies, like Goldman Sachs and General Electric, helping to prevent a deeper economic collapse while also promising substantial returns for himself in the future. He even made a late-night call to then–Secretary of the Treasury Henry Paulson with suggestions on how the US government could navigate the crisis—advice that was heeded.

Buffett's patient approach to decision-making is well-documented. As noted in *Business Insider*, he once said, "Until you can manage your emotions, don't expect to manage money," and according to *CNBC*, he once said, "I . . . make less impulse decisions than most people in business."

KEY INSIGHTS

PERCENT OF POPULATION	47
TRADEMARK	A gradual knowing
LOOK FOR	What feels true over time, a growing sense of alignment and peace about a decision
GIFTS	Gaining clarity about a potential opportunity or relationship by sleeping on it, making decisions from a place of inner calm
CHALLENGES	Acting on impulse, making decisions based on fleeting emotions, backing out of commitments, rushing into decisions and causing chaos within yourself and your environment, indefinitely delaying decisions
RELATIONSHIP NEEDS	Patience, no pressure to decide quickly, understanding that your first words may not be final, freedom to feel your feelings and to change your mind, space during emotionally charged conversations

His ability to make decisions from a calm, centered state, rather than a momentary high or low, is a perfect example of following his Emotional Authority.

At Work

We live in a world where there's a lot of pressure to have answers and to have them right away. Nonetheless, as someone with Emotional Authority, you are not meant to operate like this.

In an ideal world, you can sleep on decisions and take your time to feel into opportunities before saying yes. You may have an instinct or initial gut feeling, yes, but you are still not meant to be spontaneous and jump into a decision in the moment. The opportunities that are right for you are those you love over time, not just on the spot.

In practice, this means paying attention to your first instinct about a decision and then checking back after a couple of days to ensure your excitement persists. Waiting one to three days is often the perfect amount of time because it gives you ample space from your initial instinct.

Rather than observing a decision through a narrow lens in the moment, space allows you time to pull back and see the full picture, which gives you the perspective necessary to make the right choice. It helps you ride out your emotions, feel all the possibilities, see the opportunity more holistically, and confirm your initial instinct before moving forward.

Stepping away from a decision also ensures you act at the opportune moment. It's easy to fear opportunities will disappear if you wait. However, usually only the wrong ones do, whereas the right ones tend to get better, and your involvement becomes more enticing to potential collaborators as time goes by. So, sleeping on a decision not only brings you clarity but also tends to create (and perhaps even improve!) the timing and circumstances.

One client shared how a coach advised her to quit her job the moment it stopped feeling right. However, remembering her Authority, she chose to wait. While waiting, she received an unprecedented bonus—something that had never happened in her six years with the company. When the timing finally felt right, she gave her boss two months' notice to find a replacement. She left on good terms, and a year later, the company reached out to ask her for help with a grant just when she was looking for additional income. She sat with the opportunity and said yes after a few days of it feeling correct. Now, she works there two days a week and receives exceptional pay. Not only did things work out perfectly thanks to her patience but unforeseen opportunities also arose.

Stepping away from a decision also brings you a sense of calm. Those with Emotional Authority naturally experience emotional highs and lows without always knowing why. This means it is important that you don't make decisions in the midst of one of these highs or lows or when you're otherwise in your feelings. If you do, you may find yourself tempted to say yes during an emotional high when everything looks great only to regret it the next day. Similarly, you may be tempted to say no if you're feeling melancholic and low even though the decision could feel exciting the next day. Feeling emotional intensity or nervousness is simply a signal to pause and feel your feelings rather than an indicator to move forward with a decision.

You may find it difficult to resolve challenges with others when you are in an emotionally charged state. Let's say you're feeling upset because of a disagreement with a colleague. Rather than trying to settle the argument in the moment, let your colleague know you need some time and space, and you'll check back in once you're feeling clear. This prevents you from saying something you might regret or agreeing to a commitment that may not feel right in the long run.

As someone with Emotional Authority myself, I have personally found that when I enter into commitments from a highly emotional place, I am riddled with uncertainty and doubt for the duration of the experience. However, when I give myself time before committing, a sense of clarity, calm, and peace accompanies me throughout the experience, and I feel equipped to navigate the waves and challenges that arise. So, for as challenging as it can sometimes feel to wait, I've found it's always worth it; time brings me a calm clarity that cannot come from an outside source.

The aim is not to achieve absolute certainty in your decisions but a comfortable 80 percent level of confidence. You may not be *as excited* as you were when an opportunity was first presented because you've now felt into all the possibilities of that opportunity—both good and bad—but if it continues to feel predominantly good, you can feel comfortable moving forward. Case in point: one client chose to pursue acting because her passion for it kept returning no matter how hard she tried to ignore it. It was not a momentary thrill; it was persistent. She finally committed when she realized it always felt exciting, even in her lowest moments.

Taking the time to achieve clarity is most important when it comes to big decisions, like choosing a new job, client, or office. For day-to-day decisions that require a time-sensitive answer (like where to eat lunch with a client, what task to focus on this afternoon, and so on), it's often fine to go with what feels good in the moment, though I've personally found that taking a pause can be supportive even in the small decisions. For instance, if you receive an email from a client expressing disappointment, step away from your computer and take a walk rather than replying immediately. You'll likely respond more thoughtfully once you've regained perspective and feel centered.

However, avoid using time as an excuse to indefinitely delay decisions or actions instead of embracing the clarity that comes after a few days. I once had a client tell me she was waiting for clarity to pay her taxes. It can be easy to use time as an excuse, but that's not the point; the point is simply to give your feelings a moment to settle before saying yes and acting.

You will recognize a yes because it feels calm, clear, and settled. Any nervous energy has dissipated, and you're no longer wrestling with the decision in your mind; it just feels right and resonant. Your knowing is steady. The decision feels inevitable, like a cloud has lifted and the fog has cleared. What seemed like a question has become an obvious choice. A no feels like persistent doubt or unease. You feel unsettled. Any initial excitement fades quickly and is replaced by indifference or reluctance. As one client aptly put it, "If my feelings are extreme in any way, I know to wait."

Know that this Authority does not mean you must move slowly in general. Once you are clear that an opportunity is right and you have taken a beat to feel into it, you can be an absolute powerhouse when it comes to making that thing happen. Waiting simply ensures you enter into the *right* commitments and says nothing about the speed with which you can act once you're clear on the direction forward.

Worth the Wait

It was 2017, and I felt lost. I was building a Human Design business, but it seemed like few cared about this new modality that I knew could change lives. I was confident that would change, but I wasn't sure it would be anytime soon. Financially, I was barely scraping by.

During this period of uncertainty and questioning, a real estate developer in New York City reached out for a Human Design session for him and his partner. He was floored by our conversation and the insights it offered. A month later, that same real estate developer unexpectedly attended a retreat I hosted.

After the retreat, he invited me for coffee and asked if I would lead programming for a new high-rise co-working space he was opening in the city. He knew nothing of my professional background and didn't request a resume; he simply appreciated how I brought people together and sensed I was right for the job.

My first instinct was to say no. Although my business wasn't yet successful, my passion for sharing Human Design was still burning, and I didn't want to give up on my business partner at the time or my dream. I was convinced that saying yes meant saying no to Human Design forever.

A past version of myself might have gone with my immediate instinct. But instead of deciding on the spot, I asked for more time as my Emotional Authority advised.

With time, I came to realize something important. When I put aside the belief that taking the job meant I was giving up on Human Design, having a steady income with a supportive boss who felt like my champion brought me relief. My whole body relaxed with the prospect, and as each day passed, I felt more and more open to the idea.

The fear that I was giving up on Human Design didn't disappear, but I knew the fear wasn't the right place to choose from. The peace and calm in my body told me otherwise.

And the best part is that time for reflection helped me recognize my worth as a candidate. A week later, I met with the founder. I shared my interest in the position but proposed a change in title and salary, and I was forthright that Human Design was still my passion.

He agreed to all of it.

Time not only brought me a calm conviction about the opportunity, but it also led to a far better offer. I had always heard this would be the case with my Authority, but this was the moment I began to trust it.

And this job—the one that didn't make sense but felt right—turned out to be one of the best career decisions I could have made. The role that I thought meant abandoning my dream ultimately breathed life into it.

Four months later, with the support of my boss, I launched my own Human Design practice on the side. It grew organically as I continued pouring my energy into the co-working space, and I only left that full-time job once the Human Design business I was building outgrew it.

When you align with your Authority, you can rest easy knowing that your career will unfold in unforeseen ways that don't always make sense in the moment. An opportunity may feel right even if it appears to pull you away from your calling. All the while, it's likely drawing you closer.

In Relationships

As with career, you are meant to take your time entering into new relationships. Clarity isn't supposed to be immediate; it develops over time as you give yourself a chance to feel into someone during your highs and lows and everywhere in between. If a relationship is right for you, the feeling will persist—and likely grow.

How Do You Choose?

So, embrace courtship when exploring new romantic relationships. Don't feel pressured to reach clarity as quickly as others, even if they're immediately sure you're the one. Take the time you need to see if you feel the same. Pay attention to your initial instinct, then give it days, weeks, or as long as you need to see if your feelings remain consistent or fluctuate. Do you feel more certain about the relationship as time passes, or more doubtful? Do you feel enthusiastic about the person in different settings and at different times of day?

One client shared, "All my rushed relationships didn't turn out well, but the ones I took my time with—feeling into every step, from the first date to the first kiss to living together—were the most beautiful. Slow and steady is my jam." Another shared, "Observing whether the lit-up feeling lasts was the discernment hack my whole life needed."

While patience is required at the beginning of a new relationship, it does not mean your relationship will necessarily progress slowly. One client shared that she and her partner worked next to each other for two years before dating, and took their time to feel certain about their connection. But once they were clear, they moved from dating to marriage to parenthood within two years. They recently celebrated their fifteenth wedding anniversary.

This principle applies to friendships too. You might feel excited when meeting someone, but then the excitement dwindles, or maybe it increases with each subsequent meeting. Whatever direction the barometer moves, stay attuned to which feelings remain consistent over time. One client shared that, while she often clicks with people quickly, she has learned to let relationships develop slowly. She credits her many meaningful long-term friendships to this approach.

A relationship is worth pursuing when it feels predominantly good over time. Your conviction grows steadily. You're choosing the commitment from a calm and clear place, not from an emotional, nervous, or pressured state. In contrast, when your feelings fluctuate daily, your initial enthusiasm fades quickly, there is persistent turbulence, and you feel rushed to make decisions faster than feels right, it's a sign the relationship or timing is not for you.

You can feel most supported in a relationship when someone gives you ample space to process your feelings without pushing you to make sense of them right away. Ideally, they check in with you to see how your feelings are evolving and understand that what you say in the moment isn't necessarily your final answer. As one client put it, "I wish more people knew that I go through a roller coaster of emotions before I declare my final position. I've been pigeonholed by early reactions and had to lash out to break free from it."

It's essential to give yourself—and for others to give you—the freedom to let what was once a yes to turn into a no over time, or vice versa. Instead of seeing these fluctuations as a personal failure, recognize them as a result of not honoring your decision-making process. Giving yourself more time at the start prevents you from feeling flaky if you must back out of a commitment or relationship you already said yes to. Even if you commit too quickly, always give yourself permission to change your mind. Staying engaged in something you don't have the energy or excitement for helps no one, and it's important those close to you understand this.

In a supportive relationship, you can express your changing feelings openly, feel no pressure to choose quickly, and can talk things out without needing to have an immediate answer. One client knew her partner was the one when she realized discussing choices with him always made her feel calm and centered, rather than pressured or rushed. Even when you feel pressure to act fast, whether from internal or external sources, those close to you should remind you to take it slow and proactively build time into your collective decision-making process.

This doesn't mean others in your life won't have immediate clarity— but it does mean that they shouldn't expect the same from you. They understand that the depth of knowing that comes with time for you is worth the wait. One client shared how her boyfriend knew he wanted to pursue a relationship on their first date. It took her a month to decide. Before learning about Human Design, she questioned how he knew so fast. Now, she understands he was honoring his process, just as she was honoring hers. Another client described how supported she felt when her son noticed her feeling low and suggested she go for a run to process her emotions rather than make a decision while in that emotional space. Her nervous system relaxed when she released the pressure to know and, instead, just allowed herself to feel.

Similarly, you should feel free to take space when emotions run high. One client shared that she used to make dramatic decisions, like breaking up with her boyfriend in the heat of the moment, only to regret it the next day. She would then feel too embarrassed to reverse her decisions even when she realized they were mistakes. She ultimately came to realize that stepping away from a situation rather than making a proclamation that feels true in the moment gives her space to get clear and for her emotions to stabilize. Otherwise, acting rashly can create inner chaos that spreads outward. In my own marriage, I've noticed that I often make intense statements in the moment when I'm caught up in my emotions, only to disagree with myself minutes later. Instead of forcing myself to speak my truth immediately, I now step away and let clarity come gradually, knowing it's hard to find in the throes of emotion. Another client shared that after a tough week at work, she felt uncertain about her new romantic relationship. Instead of making a hasty decision, she gave herself time to understand her conflicted feelings. Within days, she realized her work stress was coloring her feelings about the relationship. It was her disappointment with work that made her doubt the relationship, not the relationship itself. Time brought her the clarity she sought. A Greek proverb sums up this Authority perfectly: "One minute of patience, ten years of peace."

The Cost of Rushing

When Sophie met Jim, their chemistry was electric. By their second date, Jim was already talking about moving in together. Both his conviction and the future he imagined for them drew Sophie in and made her eager to say yes. After years of searching for the one, she felt thrilled to have finally found him.

But as the weeks passed, Sophie's certainty began to wane. Meanwhile, Jim's emotional intensity never settled, which left her feeling on edge. She hoped these were just growing pains and things would improve.

But they didn't. That's when Sophie and I met.

Sophie looked worn out as we sat across from one another. "I thought I had found the one, but now I'm not so sure," she said. "Our lives became entangled so quickly. He stays at my place most of the time. I introduced him to my community, and we're already looking for apartments. It's starting to feel overwhelming, and I'm wondering if my intuition about Jim was off."

As someone who shared Sophie's Emotional Authority, I empathized with the turmoil she was feeling.

"Sophie, your initial instinct wasn't necessarily wrong," I said. "But you need a buffer period—whether it's days, weeks, or months—to confirm that instinct. It's easy to see someone through rose-colored glasses when you're on an emotional high, but time offers a clearer vision of whether someone is truly right for you. What I'm hearing is that, with time, you're not sure Jim is the one."

While my words were hard for Sophie to hear, they also offered her comfort. She realized her inner compass wasn't broken; she just hadn't given herself enough time to get clear. Soon afterward, Sophie ended her relationship with Jim. His behavior during that period only further confirmed that he wasn't the one for her.

The relationship taught her an important lesson: taking more time at the outset could prevent the chaos of rushing into a relationship and the guilt of calling it off. Sophie now understands that the true test of a relationship is how she feels about someone over time.

Practices

If you often rush into decisions only to regret them later on down the line, these practices will introduce a new way of making decisions that will bring you not only more clarity but less turmoil. If you're already comfortable taking your time with decisions, these practices will help you maintain that patience, even when you feel the pressure to choose quickly.

1. **Build in a buffer time of one to three days before making a new commitment.**

    If you tend to impulsively leap into commitments, practice giving yourself a beat before saying yes. Pay attention to your initial instinct about a decision, and then pause. Set a reminder to reassess the opportunity twenty-four, forty-eight, or seventy-two hours later. Does it still excite you? Or have you not given it much thought? Have your feelings shifted to indifference?

    You can remind friends and potential collaborators that you only want to commit to a decision if you are absolutely sure it's right for you and that time will provide you with that clarity. Taking time is not only a token of respect for you and your process but also for any other parties involved. You can convey this by saying something as simple as "I'll let you know tomorrow," "I need twenty-four hours," or "Let me take some time to make sure it feels right."

    No action is required during this waiting period. The aim is simply to observe any changes in your feelings about the decision over time.

2. **Get creative when you're feeling emotional.**

    When you're in the depths of your emotions, often the best thing you can do is let your emotions flow rather than allowing them to stay stuck and unexpressed.

    In these moments, your job is not to find answers; it's simply to feel. Engage in a creative activity like painting, dancing, or writing to let your emotions move without trying to resolve the quandary or situation at hand. You may find that allowing yourself to feel your emotions brings you to clarity more naturally than trying to seek answers or suppress your feelings.

How do you feel once you've allowed yourself to fully experience your emotions? Does clarity come more easily?

3. **Take a time-out during an emotionally intense conversation.**

   To avoid saying something you'll regret or making a commitment you'll want to back out of later, recognize when you're in the heat of your emotions and give yourself a time-out instead of responding immediately. This could mean leaving the room for a moment or asking to revisit the conversation later that evening or the next day. Remember, your in-the-moment feelings do not always reflect your true feelings. Let others know it's not about avoiding the conversation but about giving yourself space for your feelings to become clear.

   With time, your feelings will rearrange, settle, and come into focus. Your most effective communication comes from a cool, calm state rather than a hot, reactive one.

Journal Prompts

Do you tend to rush into decisions or take your time? Which approach works better, and why?

Do you fear opportunities will disappear if you don't immediately say yes? How have your life experiences validated or challenged this belief?

Does your work demand quick decisions? How does that feel, and how does it compare to environments with less pressure?

In which relationships do you feel free to change your mind? How does that freedom feel, and do you want more of it? Why?

Do you often regret what you say in the heat of the moment? If so, how could you handle emotionally charged conversations more skillfully?

Splenic

IN 2019 TAYLOR SWIFT WAS ARGUABLY THE BIGGEST SUPERSTAR IN the world. She had sold an estimated fifty million albums and grossed $935 million from her tours. She was unstoppable. And then, her former record label sold the rights to six of her seven albums to Scooter Braun, a titan in the recording industry with whom Swift had a tumultuous relationship.

After unsuccessfully trying to block the sale of her master recordings, Swift took a bold, unconventional step: she decided to *rerecord* all her previous albums to regain control over her music. Despite facing tremendous headwinds and industry backlash, she trusted her instincts.

In an interview with *Billboard* magazine, she explained, "The biggest crossroads moments of my career came down to sticking to my instincts when my ideas were looked at with skepticism. . . . We have to take strategic risks every day in this industry, but every once in a while, you have to really trust your gut and take a flying leap."

Rerecording her albums was a massive undertaking, but her new versions quickly began to surpass the original recordings on the charts, even though everyone told her it had never been done successfully before. She credits that one intuitive decision for changing her life.

In that moment, Swift trusted her intuition without pause, the signature quality of someone with a Splenic Authority.

KEY INSIGHTS

PERCENT OF POPULATION	11
TRADEMARK	Strong, clear intuition
LOOK FOR	A subtle yes or immediate resonance when something appears in your life
GIFTS	Making quick, spontaneous decisions by listening to the whisper of your intuition in the moment, the capacity for instantaneous clarity
CHALLENGES	Not acting on your intuition right away, not taking enough alone time to connect with it, overthinking, feeling it's irresponsible to act quickly, facing doubts from others about your intuition's guidance
RELATIONSHIP NEEDS	Respect for your intuitive clarity, no pressure to justify your intuition, freedom to act quickly, ample alone time to recharge and reconnect with yourself, appreciation for your spontaneity and speed

At Work

With Splenic Authority, you are designed to rely on your intuition in the moment when considering new career opportunities, often without a clear picture of where your instinct will lead you. Your intuition tends to show up as a swift, quiet certainty that something is right for you—or not—without a logical explanation. It's subtle and instantaneous.

The moment a new opportunity arises—whether it's a job offer or an introduction to a prospective collaborator—you'll experience an intuitive whisper letting you know whether to pursue it. Ideally, the moment you feel your intuition is the moment you take action. Know that your intuition may flash momentarily and vanish just as quickly. The key lies in forging a deep connection with your intuition so you can hear it when it arrives. The old adage of "sleeping on a decision" simply doesn't apply to you. In your case, delaying action can lead to overthinking and distance you from your first and best instinct. Or you may act on your intuition days after you initially felt it, when the moment is no longer opportune.

Your intuition not only lets you know what opportunities are right but also alerts you to the right timing to pursue them. One client shared with me, "I have made all of the major decisions in my life—about schooling, relationships, moves, and jobs—based on flashes of instinct in the moment that I acted on quickly. For years I thought I was just a spaz even though my life has worked out despite my deeply nontraditional path. Sometimes it's a physical feeling, and sometimes it's a weirdly prophetic little voice that whispers in full sentences."

Following such intuitive hunches tends to pay off across the board, regardless of how random they seem or the leap of faith they require. A client of mine had a sudden urge to visit the gym twice in one day. The instinct seemed crazy, but she followed it. Upon that second trip to the gym, she met a basketball coach who was so impressed by her skills that he invited her to coach his team—an opportunity she'd dreamed of for years. Another client quit her job without a backup plan. While working various part-time jobs, she felt drawn to an office and asked if they were hiring. As it turned out, they were, and she ended up working there for seven years before using that job as a springboard for her current career. One more client, a software engineer, received an offer to play keys on a national musical tour, which required her to quit her job and move within two weeks during the pandemic. Trusting her intuition, she uprooted her life and has been freelancing full-time in musical theater ever since. She recently made her Broadway orchestra debut!

As a fast decision-maker, it's natural that what feels right for you will evolve over time. While your intuitive sense about a decision may shift because the context and timing have changed, your intuition is a constant companion and will always return. If you don't hear or act on your intuition the first time, consider it a gentle reminder to listen more closely the next time.

You might feel lonely if you expect everyone to understand why your intuition is pointing you in a certain direction, especially when it's a path that surprises even you. Even then, you should follow your intuition, regardless of whether or not others understand or agree—just as Taylor Swift did when she invested time and resources into rerecording six albums based on an instinct. Keep in mind, however, that not everyone will match your rapid-fire pace of decision-making. While instant clarity is one of your gifts, it's rare and not shared by many.

To stay connected to the subtle pull of your intuition, it's vital to get still and calm enough to hear it. Invest in practices that quiet the noise and tune you into the voice of your intuition, and take space from others when you need to disconnect from their feelings and reconnect with your own. As spiritual teacher Ram Dass says, "The quieter you become, the more you can hear." You'll often find it easiest to connect with your intuition when you're centered and in the solitude of your own energy, especially in the early stages of building a connection to your intuition.

A yes can feel like a resonance, a soft voice, a gentle affirmation, or an immediate sense that something is right. It might be a nervous excitement, tingles, butterflies, an *aha* moment that takes over your whole being, a sense that there's no other option to be chosen but this one, your sight suddenly becoming clear, a gentle pull, or a click-in-place feeling in your body.

A no can feel like a lack of resonance, a sense of unease or lack of safety, a sensory mismatch like an odd taste or smell, an instant sense that something is not right when presented, an excitement about the opportunity when you're around others but an absence of enthusiasm when you're alone, or a need to justify the choice.

If you try to explain the whisper of your intuition to others (or even to yourself, for that matter), you may find yourself spiraling into self-doubt and confusion. Remember, your intuition cannot be rationalized. It is meant to be trusted rather than fully understood and is designed to guide you in the best direction in your career one decision at a time. When you learn to find quiet in a loud world and develop faith in the gentle nudge of your intuition, you can move forward with trust that you're on the right path, building what author Rachel Botsman calls "a confident relationship with the unknown."

Analysis Paralysis

Jade was at a crossroads when we met. Though she was a seasoned entrepreneur with several thriving companies under her belt, she suddenly found herself lacking inspiration and direction, unsure of which new ideas to chase. The ease and clarity with which she had previously launched ventures seemed to have vanished, which left her questioning her future as an entrepreneur and contemplating whether it was time to step away from this path altogether.

"What feels different this time?" I asked.

"I'm overthinking everything. Before launching my previous companies, I had no reputation. I was a first-time entrepreneur and felt free to experiment. I tried whatever came to me without worrying about what others thought—I trusted myself. This time, people know me. They expect success. And I'm finding myself stuck in my head, picking apart every potential idea and ultimately talking myself out of everything."

"That makes a lot of sense." I nodded.

I shared with Jade that she was meant to follow her spontaneous, immediate instinct when assessing new opportunities. The more she waited and questioned her initial instinct, the more full of uncertainty and hesitation she would become.

Jade laughed. Upon reflection, she realized that her most successful ventures were those she had instinctively pursued without hesitation. The difference now was that a newfound sense of pressure had led her to deliberate on her ideas to ensure they were perfect, which caused her to hesitate and prevented her from taking action. Hence, the stuckness and indecision she now found herself mired in.

"I've known the right approach all along. I just lost trust in my process," she realized.

Precisely.

Jade broke free by choosing to trust her instincts again, now consciously applying a strategy that had previously been her default.

Soon after our conversation, Jade sent me a note. A new business idea had arrived . . . and this time, she was running with it! Just like that, her entrepreneurial journey began again.

In Relationships

As with your career, you may find you often have an immediate instinct when meeting someone. Unlike the visceral gut feeling experienced by those with Sacral Authority, your instinct might manifest as a quiet knowing or a voice whispering that someone will play a significant presence in your life. It could be an instant feeling of comfort and safety, a flutter of excitement that draws you closer, or an unexpected calm in their presence. Not every flash of intuition will draw you closer though; some will quietly signal that a person is not for you, like an inexplicable sense that something is off. One client shared, "My intuition is a quiet nudge. Sometimes, it comes as a quick few words in my mind, whereas other times, it simply feels like the gates are either opened or closed to something. But usually, it's a nudge. It sits deeper than my emotions and much deeper than my anxious, swirling thoughts. It has come to be the ground I stand on."

Your immediate feeling serves as a beacon for knowing who to engage with, whether in friendship or romance. This might mean diving into a relationship as soon as your intuition gives you the green light, though it *doesn't* necessarily mean the other person will be on the same timeline. You may know the relationship is right before they do. For example, one client knew she wanted to make her now-husband her best friend from the moment they met. And she did. They were best friends for two years before dating for nine years and then, as she puts it, committing to be best friends forever at their wedding. Trusting your instinct doesn't always mean telling someone they are your soulmate, even if you know they are. It could just mean pursuing the relationship, confident that your intuition is guiding you in that direction for a reason. Another client felt an immediate resonance with a barista at a coffee shop. Trusting her instinct, she struck up a conversation without needing to understand why. Over time, he became a friend and eventually introduced her to her future husband.

Similarly, if you're on a date or exploring a friendship and something feels off, it probably is. Rather than waiting to find out what's wrong, trust your instinct and move on. These are not feelings to push through; they are feelings to listen to. One client with this Authority used to believe that everyone deserves a second date—until, that is, she acknowledged she often instantly knew if someone was right or wrong for her and accepted that she should just trust her instinct. Another client often heard quiet warnings like "noncommittal" or "dead end" early on in dating. Ignoring these whispers led to wasted time and disappointing experiences, reinforcing the importance of trusting her first instinct.

Your instinct is valuable not only for knowing who to invest your energy in but also for understanding when to do so. You might sense that someone is right for you but feel that the timing isn't. Trust this too. One client immediately sensed she would marry her now-wife when they met even though her future wife was in another relationship at the time. She trusted her instinct while also recognizing that the timing wasn't yet right. After that relationship naturally ended, they started dating and eventually got married.

When a relationship is right, you'll feel a clear knowing, both in someone's presence and on your own. As someone sensitive to others' feelings, it's easy to get swept up in someone else's excitement, especially when they're enthusiastic about a relationship with you or a particular choice. Staying connected to your intuition may sometimes require stepping away from certain people and spaces. It may also be helpful to make it a habit to follow intense conversations with alone time to tune in. If you discussed a big decision, how do you feel about it now, away from their energy? What feels like the right next step when you're by yourself? This is a simple yet potent practice to ensure your decisions are guided by your intuition, not influenced by others' strong emotions.

If your instincts suggest a shift is necessary in an existing relationship, listen to that too, even when it's hard. Trusting a subtle sense without an obvious reason may be challenging, but your gift of in-the-moment intuition requires it. A brave decision now will benefit your future self.

You are best supported in relationships by those who respect your instant clarity without asking you to move slowly or explain your intuition. One client shared how her husband, who has this Authority, advised her not to drive her scooter home because he had a bad feeling. Trusting his intuition, she didn't question it or ask him to explain why; she simply listened. It turned out a bad accident had occurred along her usual route. Another client, while traveling overseas with a friend, had a sudden urge to change their long-standing plans and visit a different city. Her friend embraced the adventure, and they ended up having an unforgettable time, meeting a couple who became lifelong friends. These are prime examples of why it's important not only that you learn to trust your lightning-fast clarity in life decisions big and small but that those close to you know how to support it too.

In an ideal world, those closest to you encourage you to trust your intuition, especially when they notice you're lost in your head. They support your need to get quiet to tap into your instincts, even if it means stepping away from them. They enjoy the spontaneous, fast, and exciting nature of who you are. One client shared how her partner would gently remind her to take a moment alone whenever she seemed overwhelmed by a decision, understanding that she needed space to reconnect with her intuition. This small gesture not only strengthened her trust in herself but also deepened their connection.

On the other hand, you may struggle in relationships if your intuitive decisions are questioned by others, leading you to doubt your instincts. You may start to think your instant clarity isn't robust or deep enough and begin to overthink a decision to prove you are being thoughtful even though you knew the right answer from the start. Your instinct, no matter how subtle or quiet, is the voice to trust when navigating relationships and decisions, big or small. Your work is to honor it—even if others don't.

A Whisper of Truth

When Brandi first met Michael at a get-together with mutual friends, she heard a whisper within that she was going to marry him. She'd never heard such a clear inner voice before, but it made her feel strangely certain. Brandi was in another relationship at the time, so hearing that voice felt confusing . . . but she also knew her current relationship didn't feel satisfying. She noted the whisper and let it go, trusting there was nothing to do about it yet.

A year later, Brandi's previous relationship had ended and she ran into Michael again. This time, her instinct was even stronger throughout the course of their brief conversation. She immediately felt safe and tingles ran up and down her body. This time, Michael asked her out.

That's when Brandi booked a Human Design session with me. As excited as she was about the idea of getting to know Michael, she was also terrified. "Why did I hear a voice? Why do I feel so drawn to him? I'm nervous I'm going to mess it up. I have all these expectations, and I don't know if the voice was a fluke. Am I going to sabotage this relationship?"

Splenic is the quietest Authority of them all, which can sometimes make it the hardest to trust.

"I hear you." I nodded. "Expectations can make it difficult to be present. But you are meant to make decisions based on your immediate instinct, which comes in quick flashes. Your draw to Michael is a sign of your intuition speaking to you. Who knows whether or not you'll marry him, but it's clear there's something to explore. The intuitive draw you feel to him seems undeniable."

Brandi felt affirmed that she wasn't losing her mind—and, in fact, according to Human Design, she was on the right track.

Two years later, Brandi and Michael got married—not because she forced it but because their connection continued to feel right and her intuition continued to give her subtle nudges. She now sees what she once thought was an unreliable voice as her most trustworthy guide with Michael as proof.

Practices

If tuning into the quiet whisper of your intuition feels challenging or even out of reach, these practices are designed to sharpen your ability to perceive your intuition. For those who already rely on quick, instinctive decision-making, these practices will reinforce and sustain your intuitive connection.

1. **Dedicate time to practices that help you quiet down and hear yourself.**

   If you're feeling out of touch with your intuition, explore practices that bring you quiet and help you listen inward, whether it's time alone, walks in nature, dancing, or meditation. Time alone often offers a sanctuary from which to connect to your intuition and limit external input; it helps you sift through what's truly yours and what you've absorbed from others.

This is also a powerful way to discover how your intuition specifically manifests, because it won't appear in the same way for everyone. It could be a voice you hear, a sense, a smell, or something else entirely. It may even appear in multiple forms for you.

2. **Begin with the small decisions.**

If you find it difficult to trust your intuition when it comes to big, momentous decisions in career and love, start trusting it in smaller ways. Have an instinct to see whether a company you're interested in is hiring? Look it up. Feeling drawn to spend an afternoon at a specific café? Go and see what unfolds. Thinking about a certain colleague or friend? Reach out.

From there, start to pay attention to subtle sensations as you enter new experiences. Each time an opportunity appears, you enter a new space, or you meet a new person, pay attention to the first thing you feel. The more you tune into and follow your intuitive nudges, the deeper your connection will become, and the easier it will be to trust them for the bigger decisions too.

3. **Write down your intuitive hits.**

If you feel an instant connection with someone, write it down. If you have a nudge about a current relationship or future business idea that feels unexpected but resonates, write it down. If you feel a sudden draw to a certain city, write it down.

Even if they seem far-fetched, recording these intuitive nudges lets you revisit them later to see if they were guiding you in the right direction. Did you build a connection with the person you were drawn to? Did the nudge about a current relationship or future opportunity prove true? Did that city play a meaningful role in your life? This practice will help you see how trustworthy your intuition actually is.

Journal Prompts

Do you feel connected to your intuition? If so, what does a yes feel like? What does a no feel like?

Are you considering any new opportunities? If so, what was your first instinct when they came into your world?

Do you allow your career path to evolve as new opportunities and instincts arise? If yes, how does it feel to welcome change? If not, how might it feel to embrace it?

In which relationships do you feel free to follow your instincts even if it means moving quickly and without explanation? How does that feel, and why? If not, is this something you crave?

Have you been ignoring any subtle cues or hunches about people in your life? How might these feelings be guiding you?

Self-Projected

WHEN BARBRA STREISAND READ *YENTL THE YESHIVA BOY,* A STORY by Isaac Singer about a young girl disguising herself as a boy to continue her religious studies, she had a vision.

It was 1973. The women's liberation movement was in full swing across America. And Streisand was determined to adapt Singer's ode to the plight of women into a blockbuster film.

In her memoir *My Name Is Barbra*, she reflects on feeling overlooked and unheard as a child, and she recognized similar dynamics in Hollywood. With *Yentl*, she saw a chance to fully express herself and maintain complete creative control—writing, directing, producing, and starring in the film.

Despite being told it was impossible, she remained undeterred. In *Life* magazine, her former partner Jon Peters recalled her saying, "I'm going to drop everything and I'm going to work seven days a week and I'm going to fight on the phone to raise money, and then I'm going away for two years, and I'm going to film in a Communist country with machine guns and tanks. . . . I'm going to do it anyway."

Ten years later, she did. *Yentl* became the first Hollywood film to be written, directed, produced, and starred in by a woman.

Streisand's unwavering conviction expressed through her voice and decision to pursue opportunities that allowed her full creative expression perfectly illustrate her Self-Projected Authority.

KEY INSIGHTS

PERCENT OF POPULATION	3
TRADEMARK	Clarity through your voice
LOOK FOR	How it feels to speak or write about a decision, the natural conviction or enthusiasm in your words
GIFTS	Finding answers through self-expression, discovering your true feelings by speaking about a decision aloud with someone you trust
CHALLENGES	Silencing yourself out of fear of taking up too much space, rushing decisions, overthinking instead of trusting the clarity that comes from freely talking things through or journaling, relying too much on others' advice, feeling burdened by others' opinions about your decisions
RELATIONSHIP NEEDS	Space to talk things through, active listening and insightful questions, freedom to express yourself without judgment, gentle observations when needed, honest communication

At Work

With Self-Projected Authority, the most powerful way to connect to your inner knowing is to give it a voice. It's by talking through a decision and listening to what you say and how it *feels* to say it that your feelings become clear.

This approach is not about looking to others for advice or opinions but, rather, the clarity that emerges from hearing your own voice as you navigate through your options. Speaking about a decision aloud helps you crystallize the right direction and next steps. As one client put it, "I can feel it's right the moment I speak it." Finding your answers through self-expression might look like discussing a decision with someone you trust, recording yourself speaking aloud about a potential choice, playing back the recording to listen for passion or hesitation in your voice, or even journaling. I can't tell you how many clients have shared that they will voice note a friend about a decision only to immediately follow up with a text saying, "No need to listen to that. It turns out that speaking it out was all I needed for clarity." One client described how, in a thirty-minute call with a friend, he talked himself to the point of certainty without his friend getting a single word in. When my client thanked his friend profusely at the end of the call, his friend laughed, saying he had done nothing but listen—exactly what was needed.

As you discuss potential career opportunities, start listening to your own words and noting whether there's a hint of zeal or reluctance in your voice. Often, your voice will rise and become more animated when discussing an exciting opportunity, whereas you may notice indifference or flatness when speaking about a prospect that is not the right fit. Let go of the need to plan your words and allow your thoughts to unfold naturally without overanalyzing or justifying them. Notice how your words resonate, especially those that come out spontaneously. One client found that the key to talking things through is quieting her mind as she speaks so she can hear what she truly believes and what lies beneath any urge to talk herself in or out of a decision. Another client shared that during a job interview, she felt unexpectedly moved to ask deep, probing questions of her interviewers. Both she and the interviewers were struck by the intensity of her questions, but she had learned to trust the wisdom of her voice even in high-pressure situations. Her authenticity shone through, and she got the job.

When talking decisions through, be intentional about who you share with—not just anyone will do. You might find you are sensitive to others' energy and can quickly feel overwhelmed if others inundate you with their opinions. When seeking clarity around a decision, share only with those who will serve as a helpful sounding board. The right people for the job are genuinely curious about what you're saying, ask insightful questions, and are committed to helping you discover your true feelings by simply being present for a conversation rather than telling you what to do. One client shared that when she felt stuck at work, she would turn to a trusted colleague who not only provided a listening ear but also reflected back what she was noticing in my client's voice—whether it was excitement or doubt brewing under her words. This colleague made an ideal sounding board because she was more interested in creating space for my client to work through decisions on her own than in imposing her opinion. In my experience, you can tell when those with this Authority reach a point of clarity—you see the lucidity wash over their face midconversation and sense their relief when the answers come.

Ideally, with this Authority, you speak about a decision with others, but if that's not possible, journaling or recording yourself talking about it can help you tap into the truth that comes through your own voice.

You also have a strong, powerful sense of self, and it's important to make career decisions based on your feelings about whether an opportunity will move you in the right direction, spark joy, and allow you to fully and creatively express who you are. In other words, follow the opportunities that make you feel most like yourself. As author and philosopher Howard Thurman said, "There is in you, something that waits and listens for the sound of the genuine in yourself. . . . That is the only true guide you will ever have."

Some questions to consider when evaluating a specific decision or reflecting more generally on your career as a whole are: *Does this opportunity make you feel welcomed and seen? Will it allow your full self-expression? Is your voice valued? Does it feel like the right path? Does it make you happy? What types of work and settings drain your energy, and which ones energize you? What does career success mean to you?*

When an opportunity is right, you may feel a subtle knowing or an undeniable sense of rightness as you speak about it aloud. Your words flow smoothly, and your voice has a note of confidence. There is no shyness or hesitation in your words. Your words feel like a sigh of relief, your body softens, and it almost feels like joy coming up your throat. You're not trying to convince yourself or anyone else of what you should do. As one client said, "If I try to dispute it, I'd be fooling myself." On the other hand, when a decision is not right, you may notice yourself justifying it excessively, sounding confused and unclear, feeling misaligned or uneasy as you speak the words, or suddenly aware that you don't see a path toward genuine self-expression in the opportunity.

Colleagues or friends might misinterpret your need to talk decisions out as indecisiveness, hesitancy, or overthinking when it's simply your process. If appropriate, be explicit with others about how you arrive at decisions and share how they can best show up for you. While you may not know immediately what's right for you when an opportunity arises, you have a clear process you can use to find your answer each and every time. The key is to trust and follow it—and to encourage others to support you along the way.

Painting Her Path

Erica was struggling in her career. She sensed that her next step was near but was unable to grasp it. Despite seeking advice from friends and researching potential careers for hours each day, she remained directionless.

"Why do I feel so lost? I've looked everywhere for answers, but still, nothing feels right," she lamented, dropping her forehead into her hands.

"Have you given yourself a chance to reflect aloud about what you truly want?" I asked.

I shared with Erica that the fastest, most effective way for her to access clarity was to speak freely about the decisions she's considering with people she trusts.

The following week, Erica sat down with a close friend and explained that she needed a good listener who would also ask probing questions. Her friend was happy to oblige, and Erica called me after they spoke, overflowing with excitement. As she'd hoped, her friend asked one insightful question after another, and one question in particular about what sparked her most authentic expression unlocked the clarity she'd been seeking. In answering, Erica realized that her love of painting—a constant presence in her life—was what made her happiest and was something she now felt ready to pursue professionally. As she spoke to her friend, Erica realized that opportunities to paint had been popping up left and right; she just hadn't taken them seriously until that moment. As she shared all of this with me, her voice was light and full of conviction.

I couldn't help but smile. Erica had found her own clarity not through external inputs but simply by embracing her process and giving her inner wisdom the space to shine.

In Relationships

Just as in your career, your voice is your most powerful tool to discern which relationships are worth pursuing and to make the right decisions within them. Instead of rushing or relying solely on immediate instincts, give yourself space and time to verbally process your feelings, whether alone or with others. While many ideas and thoughts may swirl within you, verbalizing them brings the clarity you seek.

One client shared, "I need to get everything out, almost like word vomit, to identify what isn't the answer and discover what is."

When considering a new relationship, let your words flow with someone you trust and notice how it feels to talk about it. Can you be your most authentic self in the relationship, or do you feel restricted and unable to express your true thoughts and feelings? Does the relationship align with who you are and where you want to go? Does it bring you happiness? Notice whether your enthusiasm and confidence grow as you consider investing more deeply in the relationship or if you find yourself uncertain and wavering. When a relationship isn't right, your voice may sound hesitant and small.

Even if others have instant clarity about a decision or a relationship, take the time to honor your own process. Rushing for clarity benefits no one; it only increases the likelihood of entering into relationships and commitments that aren't right for you, leaving you confused and discontent once you're in them.

In your closest relationships, you are best served when people honor your need to talk things out without judgment, shaming, or impatience. They don't try to fix or offer solutions unless you ask, instead noticing changes in your tone and gently reflecting what they observe if you're open to it. The safer you feel, the easier it is for your words to flow naturally and for you to tap into your true knowing. For instance, one client was having a discussion with her partner about the possibility of setting more explicit boundaries with a friend. She found herself rationalizing why she shouldn't do so, and her partner shared that her voice betrayed discomfort with the current state of her friendship, suggesting stronger boundaries were necessary. My client journaled to confirm her partner's reflection and came to understand that stronger boundaries were indeed necessary.

Another client felt tempted to give advice to her son with Self-Projected Authority, which he was picking up on and was straining their relationship. The situation only improved when she began asking open-ended questions and offered a safe space for him to process aloud. Though his answers weren't always what she would have chosen, they helped facilitate his ability to reach the decisions that were right for him, and he became more confident, clearer, and happier. Another client shared how frustrated she used to get with her partner, who has Self-Projected Authority, because he would discuss a decision with everyone around him only to ultimately come back to the same conclusion she had suggested from the start. Unlike him, her Authority provided instant clarity. Their relationship improved once she stopped expecting immediate answers from him and instead encouraged him to take the time he needed. By respecting his process, she supported him in reaching certainty on his own, which helped him step into commitments at the right time and with confidence.

Given the value of supportive sounding boards, it's helpful to identify the most encouraging voices in your life, whether among your closest friends or within your broader social circle. One client noted that her best friends are those with whom she can have an open and honest dialogue, allowing her to process decisions and big changes aloud without feeling rushed. They ask thoughtful questions and hold space for her thoughts, trusting she'll find clarity on her own if given the chance to speak freely. Another client expressed how helpful it was when a friend asked her what drew her toward a decision and what held her back; both questions gave her useful insights and brought her closer to a resolution. While no one can *always* be the perfect listener, it's essential to have relationships where you feel free to express yourself.

Conversely, feeling unheard can signal that a relationship is not right for you. This may look like worrying that your process is too messy or that you take up too much space in conversations, even though your *aha* moments are unlocked through them. It might feel as though you're speaking different languages, or perhaps you find yourself hiding or changing parts of who you are because open communication is not a priority. These dynamics not only make you feel unseen but also diminish your most powerful vehicle for clarity: your voice.

You do not set yourself or your friends, partners, or family members up for success if you don't make them aware of your need to talk things out, both in general and in the specific moments when you need it. Let them know you need time and space before making decisions, and that using your voice is the doorway to clarity. Whether or not they are the person you talk things out with, this understanding will help them honor your process and set them up to be a sounding board in the times you need it.

Taking Up Space

Olivia felt confused about almost everything in her life when she came to me.

She was unsure if her new relationship was right for her. She didn't know whether to stay in her apartment or move. She was disconnected from her community, which once felt right but no longer did. She wanted to leave the job she'd been at for five years but was scared to do so. "I feel like I'm in my head trying to find all the answers, but they never come. I'm not sure if I'm making the right moves or just avoiding them," she said.

Given that Olivia's Authority was to talk things out, I first wanted to see if she was tapping into this practice.

"Olivia, I'm curious," I began. "According to your design, the best way to reach clarity isn't to keep turning things over in your head but to speak about them. Whether it's to yourself, someone you trust, or even in a journal, expressing yourself freely helps you tune into how you really feel."

Clearly, I struck a chord because Olivia began to cry. She shared that she loved her voice and talked all the time as a child, both to herself and to others. But then Olivia's father told her she talked too much. From that point on, she began to quiet her voice and grew insecure about taking up space in relationships and her community. Unsurprisingly, the more she suppressed her voice, the more confused Olivia became about where to use her energy. Her pathway for clarity had been stunted. As a consequence, she regularly felt unsure of what to cision or hesitation, these practices are

do next and often found herself in relationships where she felt small, unheard, and uncertain.

She felt relief learning about her design but also sadness for the years she'd spent repressing her voice. Slowly, Olivia began to rediscover the power of processing aloud, regaining confidence with each conversation.

It started with our sessions, then she hired a therapist who provided a safe space, and also reconnected with a childhood friend who was a good listener.

Once Olivia recognized her need to feel fully expressed and found the right spaces to share freely, it became clear that her current relationship wasn't right. She realized her community left her feeling invisible, so she focused on building deeper, one-on-one connections that resonated with her. As her voice grew stronger, so did her clarity, and with it came the confidence to choose relationships that truly supported her. These new connections made her feel heard and free to take up space, bringing her a sense of expansion, authenticity, and freedom she had never known before.

Practices

If you frequently experience indecision or hesitation, these practices are a powerful way to regain and uncover clarity in your choices through your voice. If you typically feel confident and clear in your decision-making, they can help you preserve that clarity.

1. Consider an issue you've been mulling over and talk it out with a friend.

    Think of an issue you're currently grappling with. Maybe a challenging dynamic with a friend, a struggle at work, uncertainty about where to live, or a romantic prospect.

Choose someone who is a good listener and makes you feel seen, and let them know you need someone to listen and ask good questions, not to offer advice. See if they are available to serve as a sounding board in that particular moment. If they are, practice talking the issue out freely with that person. Notice how it feels to speak about it aloud without justifying or reasoning your way to clarity. See what unfolds when you talk. How does it feel? What do you notice in this process? Do you feel clearer after the conversation?

2. **Explore different forms of self-expression to see which ones bring you clarity most naturally.**

Leave a voice note for a friend. Try talking a decision out with a colleague who asks great questions. Record the conversation and listen back to find clarity. Go on walks, ask yourself questions, and see what comes up when you speak aloud on your own. Freestyle. Freewrite. Write poetry.

Whatever the method, identify the means that best helps you unravel your thoughts and see things clearly.

3. **Reflect on who feels good to talk things out with.**

Identify people in your life—be they friends, family, co-workers, therapists, or coaches—who listen well, ask insightful questions, make you feel seen, and refrain from imposing their views upon you. When you find yourself in need of clarity, turn to these people rather than resort to a casual conversation with whoever happens to be around.

Journal Prompts

When you talk through decisions, how does it feel? Are you left with more clarity after, or do you often feel more confused?

How would it feel to ask someone to just listen as you share your thoughts about a work decision? Is there anyone you'd feel comfortable doing this with?

If there's a work decision you're considering, what do you feel when you talk about it? What do you notice in your voice?

In which relationships does communication flow easily? How do these compare to relationships where communication feels more stunted?

Do you feel comfortable expressing yourself and taking up space in relationships? If not, what's holding you back?

Ego

ON SEPTEMBER 14, 1994, FAMILIES ALL ACROSS THE US TUNED IN TO watch *All-American Girl*, the first major network sitcom centered on an Asian American family, starring Margaret Cho.

Margaret Cho, known for her bold comedy, began performing stand-up as a teenager in San Francisco. When ABC offered her the lead role, she accepted, despite having little creative control. She valued the security and opportunity for representation even if it meant compromising her artistic vision.

From the start, Cho clashed with the production team. She was pressured to tone down her edgy style and even asked to lose thirty pounds in two weeks. Reflecting on this, she later shared on PBS, "I was too overweight to play the role of myself, which is insane if you think about it. But I didn't know that was crazy then. I just wanted to keep my job." In her later stand-up special, *I'm the One That I Want*, she joked about being told she was "too Asian" or "not Asian enough," revealing the unrealistic expectations placed on her.

All-American Girl was canceled after just one season.

Although the show was groundbreaking, the experience left Cho feeling pressured to conform rather than empowered to be herself. A year later, she released her debut comedy album, *Drunk with Power*, and returned to stand-up, where she felt free to be her bold, audacious, and edgy self. This

KEY INSIGHTS

PERCENT OF POPULATION	1
TRADEMARK	Your strong will
LOOK FOR	What ignites your heart, makes you feel valued, and empowers you to show up fully as the force you are
GIFTS	Knowing if something is right based on your genuine desire and motivation, becoming unstoppable when your heart is fully committed
CHALLENGES	Downplaying your true desires, saying yes to opportunities you aren't fully invested in, not allowing yourself enough rest before taking on new commitments, feeling selfish for wanting what you want, overgiving
RELATIONSHIP NEEDS	Encouragement to go after what your heart wants, reciprocity, space to express your desires, no pressure to engage in experiences you aren't invested in, no expectation of constant availability, never feeling like you're too much, a helpful sounding board

return to the work that lit her heart on fire led her to become a gay icon and one of the most respected female comedians of all time.

In a 2013 interview with *Seoul Journal*, Cho shared that the most challenging part of her career has been "trusting I can do this. I think a lot of Asian American kids often don't follow their dreams, because they're really encouraged by their parents to do what their parents want them to do. So it was turning against that and going for my idea of what I wanted to do with my life."

When Margaret Cho followed her desires and made choices that gave her a sense of power and control, she exemplified what it means to follow her Ego Authority.

At Work

With Ego Authority, you are meant to be guided by your desire, heart, and intrinsic motivation when evaluating career opportunities. The right opportunities are those that your heart draws you toward and that you feel most driven to pursue. Your innate motivation, which cannot be fabricated or forced, reveals whether you truly have the capacity to show up and commit. On the other hand, if you say yes to a job, partnership, or endeavor you are halfhearted about, you can quickly burn out because your heart— and therefore your energy—was never fully invested.

Unlike most of the world, you have the gift of extraordinary willpower and can persevere through almost anything when you truly want it. Your willpower is stoked when your desires are met, like the flame that lights a fire. This means your potential at work is unleashed when you have a wholehearted desire to make something happen, feel valued, and are empowered to be yourself—just as Cho was when she returned to stand-up comedy. In other words, being driven by your desires and feeling appreciated allows you to have the greatest impact and bring full energy to your work. This might mean being well-paid or receiving recognition that acknowledges your contributions. Ultimately, only you can decide what this motivating force is; you might not know it until you feel it.

How Do You Choose?

Being self-oriented in this way is foundational to your success. Each new career move should enhance your self-worth, fulfill your ambitions, and align with what you truly desire for yourself. So, consider what you need from an opportunity in order to feel successful, respected, and taken care of. Labeling yourself as "selfish" for wanting to feel valued and having your needs met can trap you in situations where your contributions are undervalued and your needs go unfulfilled. I often find myself reminding clients that this is *not* about being selfish; it's about understanding what you want and need to function optimally. For instance, one client insisted on a four-day workweek at her new job, knowing she was more effective in four days than five, and valued having long weekends with her young daughter. Another client prioritized excellent healthcare when seeking out work because she wanted fertility treatments covered while trying to conceive. Another client, a CEO, required her employees to return full-time to the office after the pandemic, confident their presence was essential to building their new product. Having these specific needs met allowed them to perform at their best.

To be honest, I often feel intimidated by the conviction and intensity of those with this Authority. It's as if they have a powerful, almost otherworldly force fueling them, driving them to achieve great feats and show up fully when their needs are met.

With this Authority, start to pay attention to your spontaneous thoughts and declarations, like "I want this," "I must have this," or "I will do this." Even if you have been conditioned or taught otherwise, the desires you think or blurt out without thinking have a determination, conviction, and force behind them that will guide you in the right direction.

It's also important to approach new commitments feeling energized rather than drained (or with the inclination that you might become drained as a result of the commitment). Rather than expecting a consistent stream of momentum from yourself, which can quickly burn you out, it's healthy to pay attention to and honor what you have the energy for—and that will ebb and flow. Making decisions from a place of fullness and resource rather than depletion ensures you will approach new commitments with energy and enthusiasm and enter them at the right time.

A yes can feel like an undeniable desire, a motivation to jump right into an opportunity and make it happen, a feeling that the full force of your power is behind the decision, a strong conviction, a wholehearted knowing, a burst of positive energy pushing you forward, and a faith that your precious energy will be appreciated. A no can feel like a lack of motivation or desire; feeling forced, drained, or halfhearted; concern that your power and capacity will be taken advantage of; or dissatisfaction with the compensation.

When considering a new opportunity, check in on whether you actually *want* to make it happen, you feel motivated to commit your precious energy to it, there's enough up for offer to make it worth your while, you will be empowered to show up as the full force you are, and your heart is in it. As Brazilian novelist Paulo Coelho writes, "Wherever your heart is, there you will find your treasure."

The Heart Knows

For three years, Lillian was content at her job. She felt motivated, loyal to her team and the company's vision, well-compensated, and valued for her contributions. Everything about her career felt right, and she assumed it would remain that way.

And then a reorganization shifted everything. With a new leadership team in place, Lillian suddenly felt underappreciated for all that she brought to the table. She knew how capable and indispensable she was, yet suddenly, it felt like no one else saw it. Slowly but surely, her desire to show up for her team and the company's mission began to fade.

This is when Lillian showed up for a session. She had long red hair and bright green eyes that radiated a fiery spirit, yet I couldn't help but feel some of that fire had been extinguished.

"Where'd my motivation go?" Lillian asked, looking at me as though I might have the answer. "I thought I'd stay in this job for another decade, but now I'm not sure."

I was particularly excited to dive into this conversation, since Lillian's Ego Authority is rare.

"Lillian, based on your design, I'd love to explore whether it's still the right fit. Are you open to a few questions?" I asked.

"Absolutely," she replied.

"First, is your heart still in this job? Do you feel driven to show up for this team?" I asked.

"Not anymore," she admitted.

"And do you feel valued? Do you think it's a fair deal for you, or are you giving more than you're getting?" I continued.

"I used to feel incredibly valued, more than anywhere else I ever worked. But now, it's like I'm invisible, and the less appreciated I feel, the less I want to be here," Lillian confessed.

"That makes perfect sense, Lillian. Let me explain why." I told Lillian that, as an Ego Authority, she is meant to commit only to opportunities where she feels intrinsically motivated to show up and is acknowledged for her contributions. Her extraordinary willpower is unlocked through proper recognition.

If the recognition dissipates, so do her motivation, will, and desire to engage.

It became apparent that although the job was once the perfect fit for Lillian, that was no longer the case. The new leadership left her uninspired to fully invest herself as she once had.

"I've been forcing myself these past few months, and it feels so freeing to finally understand that this job is no longer right for me. I am at my best when my heart is in it, and frankly, it just isn't anymore."

Soon after, Lillian moved on from what once had been her dream job, opening herself to new opportunities that reignited her willpower—a gift that she knew lay dormant within her and was simply waiting to be rekindled.

In Relationships

When your heart is fully invested, your loyalty and dedication to those close to you run deeper than most can imagine. However, much like in your work, this level of commitment relies on feeling valued and empowered by those around you. This might come through words of appreciation for all you bring to the table, thoughtful gestures that give you space to pursue your heart's desires, or attentiveness to what you want most and a shared excitement in making your dreams a reality. It may even come as a reminder of your power when you need it most. Whatever the form of encouragement, don't settle when it comes to bringing someone new into your life. Stay connected to your heart and pay attention to whether it genuinely pulls you toward someone and if you feel an intrinsic desire to show up for that relationship.

Your energy naturally empowers others, often making you a motivational force in relationships. You have an innate ability to inspire friends, partners, and family members to believe in themselves and see that anything is within reach. One client shared that her friends had encouraged her to become a life coach for years, as she had inspired many of them to transform their lives. Their recognition drove this client to launch a coaching business that quickly took off, with many of her friends becoming her first clients. Like her, it is essential to invest in relationships where your contributions are valued without feeling like you're overgiving or being taken advantage of. Others may not contribute to a relationship in the same way as you, but they must give in a way that motivates you to engage fully. If overgiving becomes a pattern, you risk resentment and burnout.

To understand which relationships are right for you, pay attention to the people you feel compelled to show up for. Who do you desire to spend time with? Who is your heart drawn toward? Who meets your needs and makes you feel that you are both giving and receiving abundantly? Where do you feel respected and free to express your desires without judgment? Seek relationships that do more than support—they should elevate your self-belief and inspire you to dream bigger.

These questions also apply to reassessing existing relationships. If you feel your motivation waning and your heart is no longer fully invested, consider if you need to make a change—whether by setting new boundaries or taking some space. Because your energy naturally fluctuates, you won't always have the energy to show up for someone even when the relationship *is* right for you, but it's important that when the energy is there, you desire to show up.

Once in a relationship, be mindful of the promises you make, whether it's a promise to attend an event, help with a task, or even show up for a conversation. When your heart is in a promise, nothing can stop you from following through, but if it's not, your energy will drag, which makes it hard to fulfill the promise and give your best. Be honest when you can't commit to something another person wants; pushing through inevitably leads to disappointment for both of you. Only making promises you are fully committed to strengthens your self-belief as well as builds others' trust in and respect for you.

Your relationships should be a safe space to express your honest feelings and desires, no matter how big or material they feel. Because your natural wants are meant to guide what you commit to, ignoring or suppressing them can lead you to enter relationships that make you feel diminished or struggle to uphold commitments once you're in them. This can leave you feeling flaky when, in reality, you just said yes when your heart was saying no. You may also struggle if others try to convince you to commit to plans you feel halfhearted about or make decisions without consulting you.

You are best supported by those who encourage you to pursue your desires, even when they do not fully understand them. They serve as a sounding board when you need to process out loud and never make you feel like too much. They recognize the conviction in your voice when you truly want something and inspire you to follow it even when it's daunting and scary. They trust the words of your heart. In their presence, you feel valued and cared for in ways that are meaningful to you.

For example, one client shared that she felt a deep craving to spend time abroad, yet her partner struggled to understand why they should uproot their lives for an unknown future. However, for her, being supported in her inexplicable yet profound desires is what makes her feel safest and most cared for in a relationship. Another client shared that her partner was resistant at first when she expressed a career move she felt she must make. Yet with time, he learned to pay attention to the moments she used the language of need, want, must, and desire—beginning to recognize these as the moments her heart was speaking. He came to see these were the times to lean in and support her rather than try to convince her otherwise.

You'll know a relationship is right when you feel naturally motivated and excited to show up without needing to convince yourself to do so. A signal a relationship might not be for you is when you feel propelled forward by someone else's conviction rather than your own. The relationship feels unequal, and you often have to convince yourself to participate. You don't feel valued, and the relationship drains you more than it energizes you.

Stay connected to the conviction and certainty in your heart as you get to know someone and reflect on your existing relationships. Is that feeling strong and undeniable, or weak and quiet?

The Power of Give and Take

When Jill came to me, she felt burned out, and it wasn't even from work; it was from her relationships.

She had always been an intensely loyal friend, but recently, she felt like her loyalty had taken her too far. Jill was proud of how she showed up for her friends—always the first at the party, the last to leave, the person championing her friends' projects and checking in on them in tough times. But suddenly, she was beginning to feel exhausted rather than energized by her friendships. She felt unmotivated to show up with the devotion and commitment that had always come naturally to her.

When I looked at her chart, I saw Jill had Ego Authority. The loyalty, heart, and power she brought to her relationships were clear.

"The thing is," I shared, "for as much heart as you bring to relationships, it's important that you are receiving too. Your relationships should bring you energy, inspiration, and reciprocity, not exhaustion."

My sense was that it was a lack of reciprocity that led to Jill's burnout. I suggested she first step back and identify where she was overgiving, and then reflect on who she felt genuinely motivated and excited to show up for without any sense of obligation.

The relief on her face was unmistakable.

"I *have* taken it too far," she realized. "I've always prided myself on showing up for people, but the truth is that I've been finding my worth in my ability to show up 'better' than anyone else. I haven't been discerning about where and to whom I give my energy, and have been more interested in being everyone's best friend than following what I actually want."

Realizing that her need to be everyone's best friend had created an unsustainable dynamic, Jill quickly identified relationships she had never felt inspired to show up for and stepped back. She had conversations to express her needs and establish a more balanced dynamic in relationships she truly wanted to be a part of.

Jill's energy for her community returned when she developed new standards for her relationships. She rediscovered her devotion and unwavering loyalty—but now, she shared that heart more intentionally and selectively, appreciating it as the precious gift it truly is.

Practices

If following what you want feels impossible, these practices are designed to normalize your desires as a key factor in your decision-making process. For those already in tune with your heart's direction, these practices will help sustain that alignment.

1. **Consider whether there are any commitments you feel halfhearted about.**

   Are you investing your time and energy in any relationships or commitments that your heart isn't fully in? Are there any dynamics that feel unequal or where your power feels unseen? If so, take the time to consider how much energy you are pouring into that relationship or commitment and whether any changes are necessary. Does it still feel right to you? Are there boundaries you could set or conversations you could have to make it more sustainable?

   Also, consider the relationships and commitments you feel fullhearted about, where the dynamic feels reciprocal, and your gifts are valued. How different do those experiences feel? Is the energy you're investing proportionate to how you feel?

2. **Keep a list of your deepest desires.**

   So often, those with Ego Authority suppress their natural desires because they feel guilty for wanting certain things or having desires they (or others) deem too materialistic. Start to embrace your desires by routinely jotting down everything you long for. Write freely and without judgment. Allow yourself to admit what you want more than anything, no matter how wild or outlandish it may seem, and begin to concretize the things that have perhaps only existed in your imagination thus far.

   It might also feel empowering to express those desires out loud. Choose someone you trust to be a nonjudgmental sounding board and give yourself full permission to share. What do you want? What motivates you? What are your most audacious desires? Talking about your desires can help you own them rather than shut them down or feel self-conscious about them. It also sets a new standard for relationships as a place where you can freely and fully express yourself.

3. **Only make promises you can follow through on.**

   When you make promises you can keep and follow through on them, you will naturally build self-esteem and trust in your powerful capacity to make things happen and will feel good about the work you're putting into the world. And, of course, the opposite is true too. If you commit to an experience without your heart being in it, it can feel impossible to make it happen. In that scenario, you may start to doubt your capacity and may even believe you're incapable of making things happen in the way you know you can under the right circumstances.

The fastest, most effective way to build self-esteem is to be selective about the promises you make.

Journal Prompts

Can you sense when your heart is drawn toward someone or something? What does it feel like? Do you usually trust these feelings? If not, why?

Does your current work motivate you? In what ways does your career path align—or not align—with what you truly want?

Do you feel you are receiving at work, whether through compensation or appreciation, in a way that inspires you to show up? How does that affect your energy? If not, how does it feel, and is it sustainable?

Which relationships do you feel most motivated to show up for? How do they make you feel, and why?

Who makes you feel safe to express your boldest desires? How does that feel, and why? Who makes you feel judged for sharing them? How does that affect you, and why?

KEY INSIGHTS

PERCENT OF POPULATION	2
TRADEMARK	Your reflective process
LOOK FOR	The clarity that unfolds over time as you talk things through, lightness and confidence in your voice
GIFTS	Finding clarity by discussing decisions with trusted people in environments that put you at ease, being a deep thinker and treasure trove of wisdom
CHALLENGES	Rushing decisions or giving in to external pressure, exploring potential choices with those who offer opinions rather than listen, discussing decisions in the wrong environments or with too few people, depending on others for direction, overthinking instead of allowing yourself to speak freely and naturally
RELATIONSHIP NEEDS	Patience and respect for your process, comfort in expressing yourself, open-ended questions, understanding of your need to discuss choices with different people, consideration of your need for the right space

Mental

IN 2020 SERENA WILLIAMS, HAILED AS THE GREATEST WOMEN'S TENNIS player of all time, won her first title as a mother at the Auckland Classic. Two years later, she announced her retirement in *Vogue*, saying, "Maybe the best word to describe what I'm up to is evolution. I'm here to tell you that I'm evolving away from tennis, toward other things that are important to me." She had given birth to her first daughter, Olympia, in 2017 and was eager to continue growing her family. Balancing family with her tennis career no longer seemed possible.

The decision wasn't easy—tennis had been her life since she was four—but it was one she reached over time with support from those close to her.

She leaned on her sister Venus, who served as an ever-present cheerleader and sounding board. In a 2022 article in the *Washington Post*, Serena Williams said, "It's been very important for her [Venus] to be part of this. She's my rock." Venus didn't offer advice or try to influence her; she simply provided unconditional support, making sure the decision remained Serena's own. Williams also talked through the possibility of walking away from tennis with her therapist, sharing in her *Vogue* announcement, "It's not real until you say it out loud." She even sought wisdom from Tiger Woods, telling him, "I think I'm over it, but maybe I'm not."

Ultimately, Serena Williams decided it was time to move on, at least for now. Just one year later, almost to the day, she gave birth to her second child.

Her willingness to talk through one of the most important and hardest decisions of her life is a perfect example of her Mental Authority.

At Work

Your decision-making process calls for patience rather than spontaneity. You are sensitive to both the people in your physical space and the space itself. When making a significant decision in your professional life, you are meant to talk the decision out in spaces that feel comfortable with people who feel supportive before deciding what's right for you. This might mean exploring your next opportunity in your favorite café or park, specifically with people you can bounce ideas off of rather than those who offer unsolicited advice or prioritize their own opinions over understanding how you feel. Unlike people who have a place in their body to look to when making decisions, like their gut, you have a reliable, gradual, and reflective process that leads to clarity every time.

Those with Mental Authority have always felt like wise sages to me. Moving at their own pace, they are deep thinkers who contemplate life's big questions and impart profound wisdom along the way. Being a fly on the wall to their patient process teaches me so much about life, and being around them slows me down, reminding me to pause, reflect, and take my time as well.

While this Authority is similar to Self-Projected, which is all about talking decisions out with an encouraging sounding board, it's most important for you to talk through a decision with *multiple* trusted people (not just one other person or with yourself) and simultaneously consider the quality of the environment you're in while you do so. Seeking (and acting upon) immediate advice from others instead of trusting your progressive journey to clarity through a series of conversations can disrupt and disconnect you from your innate wisdom.

The value in talking decisions out lies not in the feedback you receive but in the process of hearing yourself. Instead of using your powerful mind to overanalyze decisions, talk freely and notice the spontaneous insights that arise when you walk through a decision with someone who makes you feel safe and understood. And then wash, rinse, repeat, because in an ideal world, you will talk big decisions out in a few different spaces with a few different people to see what feelings about an opportunity surface over time. Different conversations illuminate different parts of you, offering a more holistic perspective than any single conversation can. Tapping into these distinct parts of yourself is what ultimately brings clarity.

However, keep in mind that you are deeply in tune with others' energy and how they feel about the matter at hand. It's easy to get swallowed up by others' feelings if you are not careful. This is why talking decisions out with multiple people rather than just one prevents you from being overly swayed by just one person. If you're feeling uncertain or confused about whether what you're feeling is yours or someone else's, step away to journal, reflect on your own, or talk to another trusted friend or colleague to see how the decision feels in a different context.

One client in her sixties shared that, for decades, she had been calling the same four trusted friends to discuss every big decision she made. She learned that each friend brought out a different version of herself, and only by consulting all of them could she find her answer. Another client emphasized the importance of the quality of people and spaces she relied on to talk decisions out. As a young competitive tennis player, she surrounded herself with those who bolstered her faith and belief in herself, which contributed to her success and ultimate decision to play professionally. Their encouragement and positive energy inspired her to be brave and pursue a career choice that, while scary, felt right.

You might be surprised by the depth of understanding that comes through your own voice over time. When an opportunity is right for you, you will feel an inexplicable certainty as you talk about it. If that clarity remains over the course of many conversations, if the tone of your voice becomes clearer, if your words feel unforced, and if there's an energy of authenticity when you share about an opportunity, these are all signs it is right for you. On the other hand, feeling pressure or discomfort when speaking about the opportunity, experiencing a lack of clarity or conviction in your words, or trying to justify your choice are all signals an opportunity may not be right for you. True knowing comes with time for you, and the clarity and depth it brings are worth waiting for.

The Power of Patience

When I sat down with Sheri, she seemed exhausted. Very quickly in our conversation, I got the sense that this was the kind of weariness that came not from a bad night's sleep but from spinning her wheels and relentlessly working without reprieve.

Sheri had launched an interior design business a few years prior, which experienced quick growth and subsequent success. However, demand had plummeted in the past year, leaving Sheri puzzled and lost, unsure where things had gone wrong. She spent her days in a state of perpetual indecision about big business decisions, all while feeling pressure to have *the* answer. As a result, she ended up making one quick decision after another. Unsurprisingly, none of them took her business in a better direction.

I looked at her design and asked, "How does making quick decisions feel for you? Do you often know the correct next step on the spot?"

"I never do." Sheri sighed. "But isn't that expected of entrepreneurs? To act decisively in the moment and keep moving forward?"

"Not at all." I smiled.

I explained to Sheri that her strength lay not in snap judgments but in thoughtful deliberation that involved talking decisions out with trusted colleagues and friends in environments where she felt at peace. It was this process of discussion with multiple people, rather than impulsive gut reactions, that would bring her to the resolution she was after.

I watched as her shoulders sagged with relief.

"I've been under so much pressure to have immediate answers, but the truth is, I rarely know right away. Realizing I'm not expected to is incredibly liberating," Sheri confessed.

It was suddenly abundantly obvious to Sheri that this pressure to have instant clarity had led to the missteps that ultimately dug her business into the hole it was currently struggling to get out of.

After our session, Sheri's first order of business was to sit down with her team and share about her need to slow down. By slowing the pace temporarily, Sheri aimed not to hamper the company's growth but rather to stop spinning her wheels and ensure the business actually progressed in the right direction. Sometimes, we have to slow down to speed up.

A month later, Sheri reported that when she gave herself space to talk through decisions with her team and a few trusted advisors, she realized they had been targeting the wrong clientele. She knew her company was excellent at what they did; they'd simply been misdirecting their energy.

The moment the business pivoted, the entire atmosphere shifted. The team's passion was reignited, new clients emerged out of the woodwork, and the business came back to life. It turned out that taking the time to reflect was the key to uncovering the vision Sheri had long been seeking, and that finally guided her business in the right direction.

In Relationships

Just as with your career, resist the impulse to rush into new relationships or commitments inside relationships even if those around you are moving quickly. Take your time instead. Commit only after discussing the prospect with trusted people in spaces that put you at ease and after landing on an answer that feels true to you. Though your process may take longer than others, taking the time to make the correct decision from the start will save time and energy in the long run, ensuring you commit only to people and experiences you are ready to fully invest in, whereas rushing will cloud your judgment and clarity. Big decisions are not the time to worry about pleasing others or sparing feelings—they're moments to prioritize discovering what is truly best for you.

So, when you're facing a big decision—whether it's starting or ending a relationship, moving in with someone, or making a major purchase—take the time to discuss it with people who listen well. As you explore the choice through conversation, pay attention to what you feel. Do you feel light and certain, or heavy and confused? What truth begins to surface? One client shared that talking through her decisions allowed her to hear the conviction in her own voice, making it easier to move forward with confidence. Whereas when she didn't talk decisions through, she tended to get lost in her thoughts, which wasn't nearly as productive and only led to confusion and overthinking. If needed, let those close to you know you may require more time to find clarity.

Also, consider *where* you choose to talk things out when making big decisions, because space is a key ingredient of your process. One client discovered that changing her environment brought answers when she felt stalled. In the wrong setting, she felt uncertain, and her words were unclear and poorly received, but in lighter, more comfortable spaces, her voice gained new focus. Another client moved from a city that left her perpetually depleted to one across the world with a backyard and fruit tree. After the move, she found that decisions came more easily because she was finally in a place where she could relax. As a bonus, you may even meet the most important people in your life while spending time in spaces that inspire and put you at ease, like a cozy restaurant, a lively neighborhood, or your favorite yoga class.

The most supportive relationships are often with those who trust your process and give you space to reach your own conclusions without pressuring you to have immediate answers. You can be your authentic self, sharing your thoughts freely and without judgment. You like the version of yourself they bring out, and it feels in tune with where you want to go. They stimulate your mind, inspire new perspectives, and make you feel intellectually engaged and respected. Communication is easy, and your voice feels valued. They serve as reliable sounding boards, asking thoughtful questions to help you uncover your truth.

One client, for instance, supports her husband's decision-making process through a shared evening ritual of walking their dog. During these walks, her husband reflects on his day and talks through any decisions he's facing. If clarity hasn't come by the end of their usual loop, he'll ask to do another loop or two. She's learned to withhold her immediate thoughts and let him verbally process as much as he needs, respecting how vital this practice of talking things through is for him.

Not everyone you know and love will be the perfect sounding board, so it's important to have a small cadre of people you can reliably turn to when navigating decisions. These are people who love your voice, prioritize helping you find your truth rather than imposing theirs, and avoid giving unsolicited advice—just as Venus Williams did for Serena Williams and as this client does for her husband. Another client with this Authority always starts a reflective conversation by saying, "I'm not asking for your opinion—I'm talking to you to hear my take in your energy." She's found that being clear about her needs sets the stage for a meaningful interaction.

When considering whether or not someone is the right sounding board for important decisions, ask yourself: Does it feel supportive to talk possibilities out with them? Do they ask useful questions? Do they let you speak freely without making you feel ashamed or as if you're too much? Are they committed to helping you find clarity on your own, or are they subtly steering you toward a particular path? Do they respect the importance of your space and support you in finding a better environment if necessary? Trusting the power of your voice and surrounding yourself with people who value it is key to making better decisions in every area of your life.

One client shared that she has become very selective about who she confides in. She no longer discusses decisions with her mother, who tends to offer solutions rather than a listening ear. Another client was considering a move to a new city and sought a sounding board. She met with a friend who immediately shared why the city she was considering wasn't a smart choice. Frustrated, she clarified she wasn't looking for input but was seeking to discover her own feelings. Her frustration faded when she realized that her friend, while well-meaning, simply wasn't the right person to help her process this decision.

In contrast, another client, recognizing the importance of verbal processing for her niece with this Authority, is dedicated to being a supportive sounding board during her niece's teenage years. Whenever they talk, she asks thoughtful questions like "Why?"—even about something as simple as choosing an ice cream flavor. This practice gently encourages her niece to express the feelings that lie beneath the surface.

A sign a relationship or a decision is right for you is when discussing it with different people in various settings brings a sense of lightness, excitement, and assurance. It feels like there is no other path ahead but this one as the words pour out of your mouth. One client shared that she gets tingles whenever she speaks the right path aloud.

When talking about a relationship or decision brings confusion and heaviness, that's a sign it may not be right. The truth may feel muddled, and you feel unsettled discussing the possibility of the relationship or commitment. Lightness and excitement don't grow over time; instead, they fade or disappear. You might find yourself second-guessing what you say.

Simply put, when deciding who and where to invest your time and energy, first ask yourself: What do I hear in my voice when I discuss this possibility with trusted people in spaces I love?

Instant Connection

Amber and Evan instantly clicked when they met at her favorite bar. Their first conversation lasted until early morning, and they decided to meet for dinner the next day. At dinner, Evan confessed his love, sure that Amber was the one for him and ready to dive in completely.

That's when Amber came to see me for a session.

I could feel a nervous excitement tingling around her. She shared

Evan's excitement but also felt pressured to match his certainty and timeline, which was causing her stress.

Looking at her design, the reason became clear.

"Amber," I said, "some people know immediately when a relationship is right, and Evan might be one of those people. But you need time. You need to spend several days, have multiple conversations, and be in different settings to truly feel if a relationship—or any decision, for that matter—is right. Speaking about a decision out loud helps you connect with your true feelings. Your answers aren't in your thoughts but in your words."

Amber realized she had been overthinking the relationship instead of talking about it. She hadn't allowed herself to openly and freely express her feelings.

I offered to be Amber's sounding board and ask her some questions, and she happily agreed.

"Amber, do you feel truly seen by Evan?" I began.

"Absolutely, yes." She nodded. "That's why I feel both nervous and excited. I'm not used to being seen so deeply so quickly."

"And how did the conversation with Evan feel? Did he ask good questions? Did you feel like you had room to express yourself fully?"

"Yes! He was curious about my perspective and met me emotionally in a way that feels so rare."

"And what about the version of yourself that emerged with him? Did you feel connected to it?"

"Yes, 100 percent! I've felt so stagnant recently, and connecting with Evan made me excited about who I'm becoming."

With each question, Amber's enthusiasm grew. Without me saying a word, she noticed it too and even commented on how energizing it felt to talk about him. Our discussion gave Amber an opportunity to realize that so many of the qualities emerging in her relationship with Evan felt truly special. I encouraged her to continue this conversation with people she trusted in her favorite spaces. She did. A few weeks later, she reported that the certainty had only continued to grow.

Eventually, Amber decided to date Evan exclusively. More importantly, she made the decision from a place of clarity and peace, not pressure. The experience also gave Evan a front-row look into her reflective process and the tools to support her going forward.

Practices

If using your voice to find clarity is new for you, these practices will ease you into the approach. And if you already recognize the importance of talking decisions out, they will simply reinforce the habit, especially when considering new relationships and professional opportunities.

1. **Make it a practice to consult at least three friends before making a big decision.**

    Normalize discussing decisions with several people and notice the nuances in each conversation. Do you feel differently around certain people? Do some people bring out new insights about a decision? Does engaging in several conversations help you gain a fuller understanding of the issue? What common threads emerge across these conversations?

2. **Consider which people and spaces feel best to process with and in.**

    The right person and setting make all the difference. Consider who in your life serves as a good sounding board. These are likely people who listen well, ask good questions, engage with genuine curiosity, and whose presence feels safe and uplifting. Perhaps it's a friend, partner, sibling, colleague, therapist, or coach.

    Think about the places where you feel most at ease and inspired. It might be a café you love, your office or a co-working space, a room in your home, or somewhere in the great outdoors. Anything goes as long as you feel good and relaxed there. Prioritize these settings when contemplating decisions.

3. **Set clear boundaries with your partner, family, and closest friends.**

    Your decision-making process is rare, so you'll need to communicate your needs and boundaries clearly when making decisions with others, because it's likely something they can't easily intuit or assume.

    This might mean asking for a few days to make a big decision instead of deciding on the spot. It might involve setting up your friends or colleagues to be helpful sounding boards by having them ask questions like "What's on your mind?" or "What direction feels right?" It could mean asking them to refrain from offering advice or explaining when they're not the right person for the conversation— and that it's not personal. It might also look like reminding them of how much your environment affects you and asking them to check in with you when entering a new space.

Journal Prompts

Do you tend to rush into decisions, or do you take your time? Which approach feels better, and why?

Who at work acts as a good sounding board? Do you seek them out for clarity? How does talking with them feel, and why?

Does your workplace feel right? How does the environment affect your energy and well-being?

Who gives you space to process without expecting immediate answers? How does that feel? How does the opposite feel?

Do conversations with different friends spark new insights in you? What do you notice when you talk things through with one person versus many?

None

IN 2014 SANDRA BULLOCK RECEIVED AN OSCAR NOMINATION FOR her starring role in *Gravity*, a film about two astronauts lost in space. Reflecting on the experience, she described her commitment to the project as "the best decision" she ever made. So, it's hard to believe that when director Alfonso Cuarón first offered her the role, her initial instinct was to decline.

At the time, Bullock was navigating a public divorce and adjusting to life as a new mom, and she wasn't sure she had the space for another film. But instead of flat-out refusing, she asked Cuarón for a few days to think it over. As she once reflected, "I don't think we spend enough time in silence, just realizing what's floating around in our noggin." During that time, she gave herself the space to tune into her feelings, free from others' pressure, to gain clarity on whether the film and timing were right. What started as a firm no turned into an undeniable yes, surprising even herself. Ultimately, she took the role, and the rest is history.

Bullock's choice to pause and listen to her own feelings rather than outside influences led to one of the most impactful decisions of her life. It is a perfect example of what it looks like to honor her Authority, which in Human Design speak is called None.

PERCENT OF POPULATION	1
TRADEMARK	Waiting twenty-eight to thirty days before making big decisions
LOOK FOR	The clear knowing that comes when you don't rush, what feels right in your body when spoken aloud
GIFTS	Patience, landing in your crystal clear truth after taking time to feel into your options, calm decision-making
CHALLENGES	Deciding under pressure, saying yes based on a transient feeling or before you're certain, not trusting your voice as a tool to find clarity, choosing based on others' feelings or enthusiasm
RELATIONSHIP NEEDS	No pressure for quick decisions, freedom to explore choices within and outside the relationship, curiosity about your needs in the moment, a supportive sounding board, appreciation for the depth of knowing that develops for you over time

At Work

In Human Design, the Authority for Reflectors is often called None. This does not mean you lack a decision-making process; instead, it means you don't have a consistent place in your body from which to make decisions. Like those with Mental Authority, you rely on a process—in your case, waiting a lunar cycle—to gain clarity.

While many refer to waiting a lunar cycle as both a Reflector's Strategy *and* Authority, I feel it's important to distinguish between the two. In this section, we'll explore how waiting a lunar cycle specifically applies to decision-making.

In a world that values urgency and instant clarity, you are meant to slow down and take your time when making decisions; your best choices come through patience and reflection. Ideally, you should give yourself a full month (a lunar cycle) to reflect on a decision before committing. While waiting twenty-eight to thirty days for big decisions might seem mind-boggling to some, those with None Authority often nod knowingly when I mention this in sessions, recognizing that this is precisely how they operate best. Of course, it's not always realistic to take a full month to make a decision in this day and age, but the key is to make decisions at a pace that feels right to you, free from internal or external pressures.

This approach is the most important when it comes to big decisions in your life, like changing jobs or committing to a new collaborator or long-term client. For small, daily work decisions and other instances in which you don't have the luxury of time, it's best to do what feels right at the moment, as long as you're in a space and with people that feel good.

Similar to Mental Authority, as you wait for clarity, it can be helpful to talk decisions out with people you trust in spaces that put you at ease. When doing this, be discerning about who you speak with. Look for people who pull the truth out of you through the right questions rather than those who want to offer advice or have an agenda. Different people will pull out different insights within you, so speaking to various people in a multitude of spaces will allow you to experience a decision from multiple places within yourself, ultimately connecting you to what feels right. The value of a lunar cycle is that it offers you the time and space to feel into all your parts before responding. This process can unfold in many ways, but here's an example: I have a client who wanted to invest in continuing education for her coaching career. To determine which training to take, she identified the program she felt most interested in but held off on enrolling. In that time, she sampled the free content that program offered, discussed it with various friends, and checked in with herself regularly to notice how and if her feelings were changing.

Part of why it's important to take time when entering new career opportunities is that you are deeply sensitive to others' feelings and require time and space to separate their feelings from your own. If someone around you is enthusiastic about a particular career choice for you, you might unconsciously adopt their enthusiasm as your own. Or if they doubt it's the right fit, their hesitation might influence you. The best decisions grow on you over time, both in the company of others and when you're alone. One client shared that impulsive decisions never yielded the same results as the decisions she took the time to consider over multiple days, acting only when it felt right instead of feeling the pressure to stick to a specific deadline.

Because you move at a different pace than most, it is important to communicate your need for time to potential collaborators and colleagues, as Bullock did when she asked Cuarón for time before taking the role in *Gravity*. Explain that this time ensures your yes comes from a wholehearted place and allows you to bring your full energy and talents to the opportunity. A patient yes benefits both them and you. I've had many Reflector clients say yes to a job impulsively only to quit a month later when they realized it was not the right fit—and never was. Taking more time upfront saves everyone involved from disappointment.

A genuine yes to an opportunity comes from a place of clarity and calm within you, feels expansive in your body when spoken aloud, and grows stronger with time. One client said, "The decision feels simple, like it already happened, even if it took me weeks to get to that point." Another shared, "It's uncertainty for days and then, suddenly, crystal clarity." In contrast, a no often carries pressure or urgency, and any excitement you feel does not seem trustworthy. It can leave you feeling uncertain or unclear when reflecting aloud as you try to convince yourself it's right even though deep down you know it isn't.

If you remember one thing, let it be this: your clarity comes from a deep, inner knowing that arrives with time, not from a slapdash list of pros and cons. It is steady, not rushed. As American philosopher Ralph Waldo Emerson once said, "Adopt the pace of nature: her secret is patience."

A Snapshot of Inspiration

Sally was just coming off of an experience that had shaken her confidence when we sat down together. A chance encounter with a photographer who was in love with his career sparked a sudden interest in photography for her. After meeting him, she decided photography was her calling too. In a burst of enthusiasm, she purchased a new camera, built a website, and was over the moon that she had found her calling.

"I've always wanted to find that one thing, and I thought I finally had," she shared.

Yet three weeks later, her excitement for photography began to dissipate . . . and then disappeared altogether.

Sally looked defeated as she shared all of this.

"What's wrong with me?" she wondered. "I was so sure about photography, and then my enthusiasm just evaporated."

Looking at Sally's design, we discovered that her Authority was None. "When assessing new opportunities in your career, you're meant to exercise patience and give yourself a couple of weeks—and, ideally, a month—to really feel if it's right," I told her. "The right opportunities will resonate over time, and your excitement will not wane."

Sally nodded and shared that this flirtation with photography wasn't an isolated episode. She had a history of being easily inspired and swept away by others' passions, only to realize she was following the wrong breadcrumbs.

I assured Sally that it was natural for her excitement to dissipate, just as it had with photography.

"Time gives you space to distinguish between what's yours and what's not, and to land in what feels right," I explained.

Upon hearing this, Sally finally allowed herself to step back from photography without guilt, recognizing it as a momentary inspiration rather than a passion or career path that could be sustained.

"Okay, I'll give myself time, then," she said. "Let's see what truly sticks."

Months later, Sally reached out to let me know that she'd found her true passion (for now) in environmental advocacy. This time, she wasn't swept away by a lightning-bolt moment but allowed a slow realization, affirmed over several months' time. This was so much more than simply a journey toward identifying and landing an aligned career. It was a journey of finally learning to trust her own process of reaching clarity.

In Relationships

While others might instantly know where they stand, your understanding unfolds gradually over time, and you might take more time to make decisions than your friends, partners, and family. Your initial impression may be quite different from how you feel about a person or decision after a few weeks; this evolution is natural.

So, when it comes to dating or getting to know someone, notice your initial feelings, but don't base your decisions solely on this. Give yourself time to reflect over several days—ideally weeks—and in different settings. Discuss your thoughts about the relationship with trusted people who ask thoughtful questions without offering unsolicited advice. Speak freely and see what surfaces.

Ask yourself: Do you feel more connected or disconnected to them as time passes? Do they consistently energize and encourage you? Does it feel good to be around them? Do you feel at peace with the idea of deepening the relationship, or do you feel uneasy? Is there any lingering doubt or uncertainty?

One client shared the value of journaling through the early stages of getting to know a romantic prospect. One day, she might think he was the love of her life; the next, she might want to run away because it all felt like too much. Tracking her feelings over time helped her sit with her changing ones, see the consistent throughline, and make a confident decision.

Unsurprisingly, while impulsive relationships can seem exciting, they're not the best fit for you. If someone is certain about you, wonderful. However, there is no need to match their speed. Whether you take a full month or not, the key is to avoid jumping into relationships out of a sense of false pressure or urgency. When you rush, you risk becoming stuck in relationships that are wrong for you. With time, you gain certainty that your yes is coming from a genuine, sustained place within you. You may find you're far more able to be present in relationships and experiences when they are born from that kind of affirmation.

One Reflector met a man online who lived across the world. Despite the distance, they quickly got serious, and before long, they decided to meet in person. As his arrival date neared, her initial excitement turned to nervousness. Feeling pressured to make a decision about the relationship too quickly, she decided to disappear instead, choosing to visit a friend and turn off her phone until he left the country. Upon a few weeks of reflection, she realized she *did* want to be with him, after all. She reached out, apologized for missing his visit, and they began again. Today, they are married and expecting their first child. Another client broke up with her now-husband a few times during brief moments of doubt, but he always waited to see if she might return. With time, she realized he was right for her, and eventually, they got married. Yet another client found that dating her now-husband long-distance was ideal. Living on opposite sides of the country allowed her to take the relationship slowly and created a scenario where she could dip into his energy for a few days at a time followed by a built-in period of reflection. They've now been together for seventeen years. These stories remind us that the right people and opportunities often remain and communicating your need for time from the beginning can help.

When it comes to major commitments in existing relationships, this approach works too. The right answer lands once you've allowed yourself to fully explore the possibility of a decision over the course of a few weeks, in various settings, and with trusted people. This process helps you connect with different parts of yourself, see the situation from multiple perspectives, and shed external influences. Ultimately, it grounds you firmly in your own clarity. As one client said, "It just takes me more time to settle in than the average person."

One client rushed into a housing rental because his partner was excited, but it turned out to be a challenging place to live. Breaking the lease was not only emotionally and energetically draining but also costly. Had he given himself more time, they likely wouldn't have ended up in that position. Another client shared that her husband kept pressuring her for a decision when they were considering divorce. She repeatedly said she didn't know yet . . . because she genuinely didn't. Eventually, he got fed up and asked for a divorce. Although she understood her now-ex's need for an answer, it made her feel rushed, and they were both devastated when it came time to sign the papers. A few months later, she felt ready to work on their relationship, which he had wanted all along, but he couldn't wrap his head around reengaging, given they were already divorced. While she doesn't regret the outcome, she wonders what might have happened had he been more patient with her process.

Some couples notice this dynamic even in the smallest decisions. One client took an entire month to pick the right teapot. His wife laughed when recounting the story but admitted it was worth the wait—they ended up with the perfect one.

You can be most supported in relationships by people who honor your need for time to gain clarity, ideally over a full lunar cycle or more. Consider who in your life doesn't rush you—and, better yet, encourages you to move at your own pace. You might find it's a relief for your nervous system to have someone introduce a prospective idea to you, followed by a simple reminder to take your time considering your options. These people understand how their energy can influence your decisions and respect your need to reflect alone or with others without taking it personally. They ask what you need in each moment, knowing it can change day to day. In contrast, you might feel disconnected in your relationships if others don't understand or respect your process, mistaking your need for time as indecision rather than the clarity-seeking endeavor it is.

A sign a relationship or decision is right is when you've taken your time to feel into it over weeks, and your certainty and excitement have remained, or even grown. You haven't rushed into the commitment, and you feel confident in the knowledge you're deciding from a place of peaceful knowing, not pressure. You're sure your feelings are truly your own.

On the other hand, a relationship or decision might not be right when your feelings keep wavering, and you're unsure if they're yours or influenced by others. You experience turmoil, heaviness, and doubt when considering the commitment. Your voice may reflect this confusion, accompanied by a persistent sense of instability and pressure.

Relationships and experiences that are meant for you will align with your natural timing. As one client beautifully put it: "I feel more embodied and in my power when I take my time, knowing it's ultimately better for everyone when I do."

Process, not Pressure

There was a palpable sense of frustration in the room when I sat down with Chris and his partner, Rose. In moments like this, I'm always curious whether that frustration comes from a relationship that simply doesn't work or a misunderstanding about how one's partner works. Often, it's the latter.

Rose had experienced a Human Design session before, but Chris was new to it. They came to me because they were struggling with deciding whether to stay in New York City or move to the West Coast. The indecision was weighing on them.

"What's going on?" I asked. "Why does this decision feel difficult?"

I could tell Rose had a lot to share and had been waiting for the opportunity.

"Every day, Chris feels something different. One week, he's convinced New York is our forever home. Next, he's looking for places to live on the West Coast. I keep orienting my life around his most recent whim only to have it change a few days later."

Chris hadn't yet explored his Human Design, but I wasn't surprised to see that his Authority suggested he shouldn't follow his immediate instincts. Quite the opposite, actually. Ideally, he needed a month to consider all possibilities before eventually landing in his rock-solid truth. The issue was that he simply hadn't given himself that time. Meanwhile, sharing his ever-changing feelings with Rose was driving her crazy because she didn't understand his process. The frustration in their relationship wasn't the result of a weak connection; it was a simple misunderstanding.

"I'm glad you're both here. Chris, it sounds like you're deep in your process. You need a few weeks to consider and talk through big decisions like moving across the country. Until you come to clarity, your feelings might fluctuate daily. Clarity *will* come with time, but you can't rush it. Rose, you can't rush Chris's decisions either."

Chris leaned forward and said, "I've often felt fickle, but you're right—the knowing always comes. The challenge is when I push myself to decide before I'm ready, like I'm doing now."

I explained that it's valuable for Chris to talk things out as he's deciding, and that it might help to talk the decision out with other people in addition to Rose. I also reminded Rose not to take his in-the-moment truth as fact and to listen as he processed without reacting immediately. She could even encourage Chris to take his time in moments when she noticed him overwhelmed with pressure to have an answer.

"You'll know when you have clarity," I reminded him. "The work is to have the patience to get there."

They left feeling lighter and understanding that nothing was wrong with them either individually or as a couple—they just needed a deeper understanding of each other's process.

A couple of months later, Chris and Rose decided to move to the West Coast. And when they did, the decision felt clear and definitive for both of them.

Practices

If the idea of waiting a couple of weeks before committing to a professional opportunity or relationship seems daunting, the following practices are designed to introduce you to this approach and help you evaluate its usefulness. For those who naturally take their time with decisions, these practices will reinforce the power of moving at your own pace.

1. **Journal often when faced with a decision.**

    Your feelings will naturally shift over time; this is normal for you. Take the time to note how you feel about a decision on a daily or weekly basis—not by making a pros and cons list but by simply observing your emotions as they arise. Whether it's the urge to end or start a relationship or make a sudden move, jot it down. Track how your feelings evolve—what do you feel the day a decision is presented? How about the next day? Does it still feel expansive and exciting a week later? This isn't about dismissing your feelings but rather understanding whether they reflect a lasting truth or a temporary emotion. Let this reflective process help you see experientially how time can be an ally when it comes to making the right choices.

2. **Experiment with talking through a decision.**

    Sometimes it's easy to forget that you can be proactive during the waiting period to find your truth. Next time you feel unclear, sit with someone you trust who you know will be a good listener in a space that puts you at ease, and talk about what's on your mind. Don't plan or overthink—just let your words flow naturally. Notice how you feel afterward. Are you left with more clarity or less? Your voice is a powerful tool for uncovering your path, so give yourself permission to use it freely.

3. **Pause to consider if you're acting under pressure before making a new commitment.**

We often rush into our decisions, despite the fact that many of us, including you, benefit from a slower pace. If you can't wait a complete month, try to ensure you at least have a timeline that gives you space to consider a decision from multiple moods and perspectives so you can commit from an unhurried, confident place rather than a pressurized one.

When making a decision, take a moment to reflect on these questions: *Is the decision coming from a sense of urgency within you? Is it being influenced by an external pressure that's being placed upon you?* Being aware of where and from whom you're feeling pressure is a powerful tool to ensure you don't commit to the wrong opportunities from the outset. The best decisions respect your timing—they're never rushed.

Journal Prompts

For big decisions, do you prefer taking time to reflect or acting on your first instinct? Which approach feels better, and why?

Do your colleagues respect your need to take your time, or do they pressure you to make quick decisions? How does it feel to be rushed versus having space to move at your own pace?

Are you often influenced by others' enthusiasm when making decisions? How does that feel? How can you ensure your decisions come from a more authentic place within you?

Are there friends who are especially helpful when you talk through decisions? What actions or behaviors do you find most supportive?

What do you notice about relationships you've jumped into impulsively compared to those you've taken time to explore?

Conclusion

IT'S HARD TO OVERSTATE HOW MUCH MY LIFE HAS TRANSFORMED since that fateful evening in 2015 when a stranger at a party read my Human Design chart for the first time.

I made a complete career shift, built a flourishing business, married my best friend—the person who made me feel the most seen in the entire world—and started a family. I moved from the city to the woods and shifted my focus from a larger community to deeper, more meaningful one-on-one relationships. I went from feeling indecisive and unclear to full-bodied in everything I do. And that was just the beginning.

Eventually, as I began to uncover the designs of my family, friends, colleagues, and children, I noticed a palpable shift in my ability to empathize, collaborate, and connect with them. Human Design helped me remember, as marriage and family therapist Vienna Pharaon once said, "You are not me and I am not you. That one sentence can help save so many of us time and time again."

Here are just a few of the ways that learning the designs of my loved ones has transformed my relationships.

As a Projector, I've always been eager to offer advice and share what I see. It's natural for me to notice how things can be improved, and I assumed—mistakenly—that people would want to hear my thoughts right away. My sister, however, taught me otherwise. As a Manifestor, she is not here to be guided or told what to do. Offering advice when she didn't seek it only pushed her away. I learned not to offer advice unless she asked for my insight, and that small change has made all the difference in our relationship.

My dad, also a Projector, has always taken rest seriously and feels comfortable skipping gatherings if it means he gets a precious moment to himself. As a misaligned Projector, I used to get upset when he chose to prioritize time alone over time as a family. But once I understood how sensitive he is as a Projector, my compassion for him bloomed. I went from wanting him to change to admiring how well he cares for his energy. He now serves as an inspiration for what it looks like to honor our need for regular rest, space, and time alone as Projectors even when those around us don't get it.

My husband, a Generator, is the most capable man I've ever met. It's tempting to rely on him for everything, and often, I do. However, Human Design taught me that just because he has the capacity to take on all those responsibilities doesn't mean he should. Quite the opposite, actually. When he is free to pursue what he loves and isn't weighed down by endless tasks, he's happier, lighter, and more energetic. By honoring his energy as sacred and respecting his boundaries—even when they clash with my desires—I make him feel respected and supported. He's shown me that nothing beats being around a lit-up Generator.

My toddler, a Manifesting Generator, has more zest for life than I ever imagined possible. She's a walking, talking ball of sunshine, leaving everyone in awe of her charisma. Even at just two years old, it's clear she can't be contained, and I have no desire to try. Human Design taught me the value of giving her options, knowing she often doesn't recognize what she wants until it's in front of her. I pay close attention not only to her words, but to her gut responses, with the intention of inspiring her to trust her instincts as she grows. As a Projector mother of a Manifesting Generator with boundless energy, I've also learned the importance of taking time for myself without guilt.

My Reflector friend taught me the beauty of fluidity. I used to take it personally when she backed out of a commitment and wondered why she acted differently in group settings compared to one-on-one. Discovering her design helped me realize that her energy shifts daily. I learned to give her grace when she's not up for something she was excited about yesterday and to stay curious about what she wants in the moment. When I stopped expecting her to be like me or like anyone else, our connection deepened. I came to admire her greatest gift: an uncanny ability to sense when something is amiss and gently speak to the heart of it. I now feel incredibly lucky to have her wisdom in my life, as it often lingers long after our time together.

Human Design doesn't limit who we can be friends or partners with; it simply helps us be the best we can be with the people we choose.

Ultimately, our lives are a series of choices.

Should I stay in this relationship?

Should I take this job?

Should I go on this date?

Should I share my story with this person?

Should I live in this city?

Moving forward, armed with your design as a compass, you are empowered to walk a path of clarity and confidence.

So, go out there, and choose what's best for you.

Acknowledgments

MY DESIGN HAS TAUGHT ME THAT THE MORE I SURROUND MYSELF with the right allies, the more successful I'll be, and this book is proof of that. I did not do this alone.

First, thank you to my husband, Jared, for holding the vision for this book. This book is as much yours as it is mine, and no one knows that better than you. Thank you for continually challenging me to step up and grow even when it was tough and even when I resisted—which was a lot. Thank you for setting aside so much time to dive into this book and make it great. Most importantly, thank you for being the partner and father to our daughters that I've always dreamed of. You are the part of my life I never doubt.

Thank you to my clients, students, and community. Your willingness to share your stories with me has shaped this book into what it is. You've turned it from a collection of insights into a reflection of Human Design in action. While I've studied Human Design for a decade, my most meaningful learning has always come from you.

Thank you to my agent, Tess Callero, for your patience over the years until I was ready to write this book. From day one, you saw the need for this book, understood our vision, and believed in me every step of the way. Thank you for being my champion. I can't imagine bringing this to life without you.

Thank you to my publisher, HarperOne. Anna Paustenbach, thank you

Acknowledgments

for reaching out with the idea for a book, not knowing I was already working on a proposal. From the moment we connected, I knew HarperOne was the right home, and your early wisdom shaped this book. And thank you to Angela Guzman, who jumped in as a Human Design newbie, for bringing your marketing brilliance and pointed insights to make this book the best it could be.

Thank you to my book coach, Nikki Van Noy, who held my hand throughout this process, especially during the toughest moments. Thank you for falling in love with Human Design and reminding me just how essential this book is when I needed to hear it the most. I'll never forget the day you told me you now read to your young daughter about her design each day, giving her full permission to step into her Manifestor power. Your fingerprints are all over this book.

Thank you to Ra Uru Hu for trusting the vision that came through and bringing Human Design into the world. And thank you to Richard for introducing me to Human Design back in 2015, being my first teacher and mentor, and inviting me to study and share it with the world. None of this would have happened without you.

Thank you to my sister, Andrea, for stepping in at the last minute to offer your edits and brilliance to this project. I appreciate you suspending your disbelief and setting aside your hardcore journalistic background to get your hands dirty with this mystical system. Thank you for always supporting my path, no matter how far it diverges from yours.

Thank you to my team for holding it all together while I disappeared into book land much longer and more immersively than I imagined.

And finally, thank you to my little toddler for being the brightest ray of sunshine. Your presence infused joy and levity into what sometimes felt like a never-ending journey. To the daughter in my belly, thank you for taking it easy on me during this pregnancy and being a trooper through those early-morning work sessions. I'm especially grateful you waited until I finished the book to make your entrance into the world. I can't wait to meet you—and, of course, I can't wait to look up your design the minute you're born.

Thank you, thank you, thank you.

Additional Resources

THIS BOOK IS JUST THE BEGINNING.

If you're ready to dive deeper into your design and the designs of those you love, visit humandesignblueprint.com.

There, you can order a hyperpersonalized guide all about your unique design that goes way beyond Type, Strategy, and Authority.

If you're ready to go even farther down the rabbit hole, you can also enroll in our Human Design Coaching Certification, which is an evergreen online course that will make you a Human Design expert.

Web: humandesignblueprint.com

Instagram: @humandesignblueprint and @erinclairejones